BEHOLDEN

BEHOLDEN

*Religion, Global Health,
and Human Rights*

SUSAN R. HOLMAN

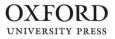

OXFORD

UNIVERSITY PRESS

OXFORD
UNIVERSITY PRESS

Oxford University Press is a department of the University of
Oxford. It furthers the University's objective of excellence in research,
scholarship, and education by publishing worldwide.

Oxford   New York
Auckland   Cape Town   Dar es Salaam   Hong Kong   Karachi
Kuala Lumpur   Madrid   Melbourne   Mexico City   Nairobi
New Delhi   Shanghai   Taipei   Toronto

With offices in
Argentina   Austria   Brazil   Chile   Czech Republic   France   Greece
Guatemala   Hungary   Italy   Japan   Poland   Portugal   Singapore
South Korea   Switzerland   Thailand   Turkey   Ukraine   Vietnam

Oxford is a registered trademark of Oxford University Press
in the UK and certain other countries.

Published in the United States of America by
Oxford University Press
198 Madison Avenue, New York, NY 10016

Library of Congress Cataloging-in-Publication Data
Holman, Susan R.
Beholden : religion, global health, and human rights / Susan R. Holman.
pages cm
Includes bibliographical references and index.
ISBN 978-0-19-982776-3 (cloth : alk. paper)
1. Health—Religious aspects.   2. Medicine—Religious aspects.   3. Health—Religious
aspects—Christianity.   4. Medicine—Religious aspects—Christianity.   I. Title.
BL65.M4H65 2015
201'.7621—dc23
2014024456

In memory of
Virginia Holland Andrews
(1915–2011)

CONTENTS

BEHOLDEN

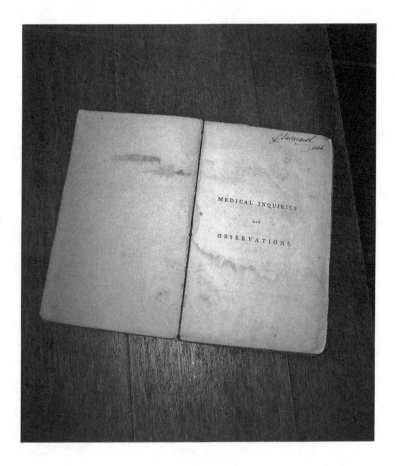

MEDICAL INQUIRIES

AND

OBSERVATIONS.

INTRODUCTION

THE SUMMER OF 2009 stands out in my memory as a long season of sultry days and nights that were brighter but no less brutal than the winter they followed. My father died in March, after weeks of medical crises and some of the worst New England snowstorms in years. The burden of his care and of settling his estate fell on my shoulders, literally, first as I tried to balance the hospital odyssey with shoveling snow, and then, in the months following his death, as I physically moved an infinity of stuff my parents had accumulated over fifty years in the same house. Throughout that time I was also working a regular job, determined in a down-spiraling economy to keep myself gainfully employed. Despite the snow and summer showers, it was a dry and desiccating year, menopausal in its emptiness. I don't remember weeping once.

As winter turned to summer, spring rushing past on a weekend of early lilacs, I spent each evening inhabiting the dust-filled silence of the late Victorian house where I had grown up. The house was packed cellar to attic, including the residue of boxes and trunks that my three grandparents had brought when they all moved in together with us early in my teens. In the simple act of settling my father's estate, as I hauled out hundreds of plastic trash bags, dragged filthy rugs and broken furniture to the curb, boxed up household poisons for the town's toxic waste disposal, and wrangled with auctioneers, painters, lawyers, electricians, and plumbers, I found myself unsettling nearly three hundred years of memories.

One evening in late July, in a room that had once been my grandmother's, I opened a small wicker trunk that, I am sure, had not moved in forty years, though I had never seen it. Nor had I seen the book that lay near the top, its cover water-stained, its spine hand-stitched, the uneven pages pressed between heavy boards. I opened the book gingerly. The paper was seamed and textured like a stiff but comfortable old cotton sheet.

July 22, 1793, someone had written on the inside front cover. Not ancient, then, I thought to myself—or not as old as some of the books and manuscripts I studied in my work on the early Christian history of religion and medicine. But certainly this book was older than my grandmother's other books, which were mostly gilded, leather-bound classics from the late nineteenth century. This book was obviously very different, prized even.

Some handwritten text on the inside front cover had been blotted out, two final words barely legible through the dried black puddle on the page: *The Author*. So, I guessed, the book had been a gift from the author. Impossible to know the first owner's name, the blot so thick it mirrored on the facing page when someone had shut the book before the ink was dry. I turned the flyleaf to read the title, the old lead type imprinted deep in small caps: MEDICAL INQUIRIES AND OBSERVATIONS. A subsequent owner had inscribed his name in the top right corner of this leaf, a name and date in an elegant hand very different from that blacked out on the previous page: *S. Saltmarsh, 1836*. And on the next page the full title: *Medical Inquiries and Observations. To which is added an Appendix, Containing Observations on the Duties of a Physician, and the Methods of Improving Medicine. By Benjamin Rush, MD Professor of Chemistry in the University of Pennsylvania. The Second Edition*. Below it was the publication date: 1789.

A quick Google search on "Benjamin Rush" and the book's title intrigued me enough to go to the library to learn more. Rush, I soon discovered, had been a leading physician in early American medicine, and one of the first American advocates for universal health care, prison reform, the abolition of slavery and capital punishment, equal education for girls and boys, and the value of respect and dignity in treating those who suffered from mental illness.[1] A signatory of the Declaration of Independence, he also founded the first free dispensary in America, in Philadelphia in 1786. In August 1793, two or three weeks after he gave this book to a now-unknown recipient, a yellow fever epidemic struck Philadelphia, keeping Rush frantically busy treating thousands of patients over the next few months. After the epidemic abated, between his teaching and political duties, Rush would continue to expand his book, focusing it increasingly on mental health. By his death in 1813, *Medical Inquiries and Observations upon the Diseases of the Mind* reached four volumes. It would become "Rush's greatest gift to medical science and greatest claim to immortality."[2]

Rush was also keenly religious. A regular presence at Episcopalian, Presbyterian, and Unitarian services, he "set the record among Philadelphian physicians for attending worship, even keeping pews in several churches simultaneously so that he might visit the nearest one should he desire communion with his Maker during rounds."[3] He described his faith as "a compound of the orthodoxy and heterodoxy of most of our Christian churches";[4] he was also sympathetic to and respectful of both Native American beliefs and Orthodox Judaism.[5] His career—and his book—would profoundly influence a number of emerging nineteenth-century Congregationalists who were finding new theological expression as Unitarians and Universalists. One of these was the Rev. Dr. Seth Saltmarsh.

Saltmarsh was twenty-five years old when he inscribed his name in the copy of Rush's text that was to make its way into my grandmother's trunk. After medical studies in Philadelphia, where he qualified as a doctor in 1837,[6] Saltmarsh was ordained a Unitarian minister and went on to preach at churches in Vermont, New Hampshire, Tennessee, and Massachusetts. Between 1851 and 1853, he served in a small Unitarian Congregationalist parish in Wilton, New Hampshire. It was perhaps during this time that Saltmarsh would pass the book on to either Dr. John Trevitt or John's brother,

Henry. These Trevitt brothers were New Hampshire physicians whose family had lived since the mid-1700s in the village of Mont Vernon, seven miles up the road from Wilton. Both John and Henry had studied medicine with their father's youngest brother, William, an 1830 Dartmouth graduate who (briefly) attended classes at the University of Pennsylvania before going West to practice medicine in frontier Ohio. The story of the Trevitts, and their odyssey into public health and international medicine in nineteenth-century politics, is told in more detail in Chapter 3.[7]

During the years when he was writing the book that would shape the medical training of so many early American physicians, Benjamin Rush had a special religious concern for providing medical care for the poor. Concluding a chemistry course he taught in February 1789, he delivered a lecture on "Observations on the duties of a physician, and the methods of improving medicine. Accommodated to the present state of society and manners in the United States." The lecture was included as an appendix in all editions of *Medical Inquiries and Observations*. In this text, Rush advised his students that:

> the poor of every description should be the objects of your peculiar care. Dr. Boerhaave used to say, "they were his best patients, because God was their paymaster." The first physicians that I have known, have found the poor the steps by which they have ascended to business and reputation. Diseases among the lower class of people are generally simple, and exhibit to a physician the best cases of all epidemics, which cannot fail of adding to his ability of curing the complicated diseases of the rich and intemperate. There is an inseparable connection between a man's duty and his interest. Whenever you are called, therefore, to visit a poor patient, imagine you hear the voice of the good Samaritan sounding in your ears, "Take care of him, and I will repay thee."[8]

Speaking here as a devout (if eclectic) Christian, Rush exhorts medical practitioners to be sensitive to the biblical paradox between gift and gain, that is, the idea that attending the poor will ensure the doctor's true profit and success. He implies that such action is not just good for the poor and the doctor, but also an expression of healthy civic duty, something that will benefit society itself, by increasing the doctor's skill in "all epidemics."

The idea that God will bless those who help the poor is an ancient and popular belief common in all three of the world's leading monotheistic religions. It may be curious that Rush appeals to the New Testament story of the Good Samaritan (Luke 10:25–37) only to advise his students to model not the Samaritan but the paid innkeeper, hardly the hero of the biblical story. And yet the innkeeper, just like Rush and his students, would have been keenly attentive to money in the economic and civic order, and to caring for the sick and weary body.

Rush did not merely spout moral platitudes. He really believed what he told his students, that the poor were his "most profitable patients, for God is their paymaster."[9] Indeed, while he was rigorous about his bills, bookkeeping, and profits, his treatment of the poor became a lifelong commitment after a dream he had while sick with yellow fever years earlier, in 1780. In the dream, he would later note in his diary, a poor woman told him that he owed his life to the prayers of his poor patients.[10] Friends remembered his last words, from his deathbed addressed to his son, as "Be indulgent to the poor."[11]

RELIGION AND WORLD HEALTH: A DISCOMFITING PARADOX?

Rush's views on religion, education, slavery, mental illness, and universal health care may have been admirable and ahead of his time, but I suspect that most health professionals today—especially those who share his "peculiar care" for the poor—would be appalled by his patronizing comment about the "simplicity" of diseases "among the lower class" and his explicitly self-serving advice that the poor provide an opportunistic stepping stone toward good business and an eminent reputation. These phrases seem instead to suggest a religious "instrumentalization" of the poor—making them into passive objects for the more powerful religious donor's greater spiritual good. Such a view is widely condemned today as a symptom of "colonialism" and a "missionary" mentality common to countries in the rich "global North" (that is, Western Europe and much of North America). This view is usually associated with well-meaning individuals eager to "help" the sick and suffering in lower- and middle-income countries associated with areas of the world known in modern economic development lingo as the "Global South."[12] The most commonly identified problem with this view is that it undermines equity, justice, and health by stratifying the capability, potential, and constructive agency of people according to historical power imbalances that have abused and subjected groups across the ages. When it persists, such an attitude perpetuates implicit biases that continue to affect health care and aid efforts around the world. As one physician active in humanitarian aid work today has put it, "There are ways of being helpful and there are ways of *not* being helpful. You can learn a lot in both situations. But in the latter, beware: you are deadening down your own sensitivity to human dignity. This has been a problem with the humanitarian community for decades."[13] My focus in this book is to reflect on the role of religious faith—chiefly but not solely Christianity, because it is what I know best—in such common tensions today, and to explore variant perspectives that could shape more thoughtful and respectful faith-based lenses for perceiving and engaging with what today is commonly called "global health" (as defined further below).

Just as Benjamin Rush's appeal to biblical imagery illustrated for eighteenth- and nineteenth-century America, religious faith has long been connected with ideals of physical well-being. Even today a high percentage (some say 40 percent) of health-care services around the world are founded and funded by faith-based organizations or initiatives.[14] And many who work in health care continue to be motivated by personal religious or philosophic values. This means that historical religious traditions continue to have a huge impact on contemporary dialogue about physical need, disease, hunger, and the potential of economic development and earning options to improve human life. Individual health behaviors are also often informed by faith beliefs and practices that relate, for example, to food, blood, purity laws, traditional medicines, and taboos. Religion influences factors such as: social determinants of health (discussed further below), health risks, and disparities; attitudes toward wealth, poverty, gender, and suffering; health-care policies; ethics and law as they relate, for example, to human rights and human dignity; and cultural history as well as historical interpretations of disease, wellness, and contagion.

Given the complexity of these connections and influences, there is no one "right" way to talk about how religion relates to health. As a historian whose work crosses both fields, I have chosen in this book to explore this theme by telling stories that offer select examples of just a few such approaches. The chapters focus on such themes as the agency of religion as it relates to certain aspects of global health; the history of economic, social, and cultural (ESC) rights; an asset-based development model; traditional ideas about charity in health relief efforts; and the role of pilgrimage, past and present. These are the topics most familiar to me, but many others might also be explored in related conversations. Through the stories in this book, I consider some of the different ways that conflicts over ideals like charity, deity, human rights, economic development models, and social justice all shape religious dialogue in the arena of health care and health-care policy, both in the nation where I find myself, the United States, as well as around the world, wherever American culture and influence intersects with other communities, ideas, and events. This is a very small book in comparison to the breadth and complexity of these issues. By touching on just a few themes, I hope the book might invite deeper conversations between persons who are shaped by religious faith or the study of religion and those in the worlds of health-care services, health policy, public health (defined further below), traditional medicine, the history of medicine and culture, and the role of health in economic, social, and cultural rights.

"I *hate* religious groups!" one emergency physician told me frankly. She spent several weeks every year donating her time abroad to provide medical care with social justice in an extremely poor community, and saw only the harm of groups that swooped into the villages she served, short-term church-based missions intent on "fixing up" and "saving" whatever they identified as problems. Her blunt and dismissive reaction illustrates the common atmosphere of alienation that often stands between religious aid workers or zealous "first-world do-gooders" and health professionals who are either local citizens of the affected communities or else Western visitors or expatriates who are trying to be sensitive to justice, rights, and human dignity. Especially since the events of September 11, 2001, the role of religion in global health has become a topic for serious dialogue whether one is "religious" or not. Within that dialogue, the complex connections and fraught tensions over differences and diverse priorities persist, even among those who might share Benjamin Rush's "peculiar care" for the poor.[15] There is a trend, for example, of short-term volunteers and students trying to prepare ahead for overseas health projects through training in what is popularly called "cultural competency." And yet even such efforts may cause problems if they are treated like a "boot camp" meant to produce overnight cultural experts. Better, says Dr. Paul Farmer and others, to cultivate instead an attitude of "cultural humility," one that focuses not on "helping" but always and above all on *learning* from those one encounters in cultures outside one's own comfort zone.[16]

ABOUT THIS BOOK

I should make it clear here that this book is *not* intended to be a practical or "how-to" guide for field-based philanthropy. Rather, the chapters will reflect on ideas, particular themes in which religion contributes to what might be called ethical tensions in global health today. As someone who works within the world of academia rather than the world of social activism or religious ministry, I tell stories about actions in order to invite readers to think more deeply about the ideas they suggest or represent, and to begin to explore creative associations that may (though they might not necessarily) lead to new or traditional but alternative ways of thinking constructively.

There is a keen need for such cross-disciplinary storytelling. Such narratives may help tease out a variety of issues related to poverty and disease that remain unresolved in world health today. This was emphasized, for example, in a recent book by World Bank consultant Katherine Marshall, who tells of a 1998 effort between global religious leaders and economists concerned with world health. When the group brought together those who funded international development aid in more than 180 countries and representatives of global religious institutions, their attempts to talk with one another and foster mutual understanding failed completely. The effort, Marshall noted, met with significant resistance despite being coordinated by the then-president of the World Bank, James D. Wolfensohn, and the then-archbishop of Canterbury, George Carey. The tensions uncovered "the perception that ethics were largely invisible" in global public efforts at economic development.[17] While this book is not explicitly about ethics as a formal discipline, it is vital to keep in mind that invisible and unstated ethical tensions and biases may undermine even the best intentions for global health efforts. Readers who wish to push beyond the narrow focus of the stories may find useful resources for further study in the bibliography.

Any book-length journey through ideas that connect both religion and health might logically begin with a consideration of *pilgrimage,* travel through and to a holy place. Chapter 2 explores this idea of pilgrimage by considering global health in the context of stories about travel that are related to a search for physical or spiritual healing. The chapter begins with my experience, in 2013, attending a Hindu pilgrimage festival in India as part of a cross-disciplinary venture in academic global health. I then reflect on related themes as they relate to ways that such transitions mark the body itself, for example through the health challenges of migration, water purity, humanitarian disasters, and bone pathology. The chapter concludes with thoughts on the shape of religion as it contributes to global health and the human rights discussion for a better world.

Chapter 3 returns to the story of the Trevitt doctors, introduced above, and the role of *civic duty* as integral to religious identity in the nineteenth-century history of public health. Through this historical journey into America's (relatively) recent past, we may glimpse what the history of public health in America meant for real people through policies and attitudes that continue to shape American health policy today. The first half of Chapter 3 draws on Benjamin Rush's philosophy on health care for the poor as it played out through the careers and health policy practices of several nineteenth-century physicians and faith/health tensions in the early American poorhouse. The second half of the chapter turns to explore in detail the career of young Henry Trevitt, his reluctant journey to becoming a doctor, including his encounters with epidemics, international political scandal, small-town murder, and his service to the local poor. Henry's career choices, his foibles, and the forces that shaped his world may also help to illustrate how many in positions of power today still continue to act and justify their actions in aid efforts related to health around the world.

Chapter 4 considers a topic that is especially controversial to many religious persons who have strong opinions about health-care policy around the world today: that of *human rights*. It is my view that "modern" human rights history and ideas should matter for people of religious faith and that anyone engaged in faith-based aid organizations has a fundamental responsibility to understand something about this issue and be familiar with resources that are available to help foster such accountability. Rather than address human rights in general—a huge topic that is far beyond the narrow focus of this book—I look specifically at what are called "economic, social, and cultural" (ESC) rights. ESC rights are those rights that are most directly relevant to concerns about religious charity, aid, and social justice. The chapter traces the history of the development of ESC rights as a formal concept—a concept shaped by people who cared deeply about religious faith—in the formation of the 1948 Universal Declaration of Human Rights (UDHR) and particularly its Article 25. Human rights play a leading role in global health efforts, policies, and practices today, and I suggest that there is more harmony than difference when we look at the underlying moral concerns and values that most directly and urgently relate to health-care equity in any society.

Chapter 5 offers a case-study-like story about a very different approach that is also common in contemporary economic efforts and faith-based aid: *asset-based community development*. The chapter traces the history of a multi-country research consortium, the African Religious Health Assets Programme (ARHAP). ARHAP began in Southern Africa and has over time improved health and health-care interventions even in poor neighborhoods in the United States. From its beginnings early in the twenty-first century, the consortium seeks to nurture collaborative relationships between religion and health care through research that looks at the theory and health-altering practices of affirming and applying *religious health assets*. ARHAP-related research—and its translation into action at the level of local communities—may offer an encouraging example of improving health and health policy at both the local and global level.

The final chapter, Chapter 6, contains the only extended reflection in the book on what we today call charity, here through the lens of the idea of the *gift*. This chapter considers gift concepts in three common activities relevant to philanthropic aid pertaining to health: economic development, religious liturgy, and the tensions between humanitarian relief and social justice shaped by the ideals of "solidarity." Charity is something we all love to hate, yet it persists as a religious ideal that inspires altruism. No discussion of faith-based responses to health can entirely dismiss the fact that charitable activities are alive and well in virtually every religious organization and culture. The chapter concludes the book by exploring the broader nuances of this traditional "gift-based" response that characterizes so many faith-based health-care services.

ON SOME COMMON TERMS

Some of the common words and phrases used throughout the book may be unfamiliar to some readers. The leading concept suggested by the book's title—"beholden"—is discussed further in the next section. But a number of more obviously health-related terms used throughout the book will also have different meanings for different people. It may be useful to provide here a brief overview of what I mean by several particular phrases: "health," "public health," "the social determinants of health," and "global health."

Health

The World Health Organization (WHO) defines health as "a state of complete physical, mental and social well-being and not merely the absence of disease or infirmity."[18] This definition describes what is obviously an ideal. This ideal is one that often shapes how we live and may use the health-care services that are available to us. It is important to keep in mind that the WHO definition of health does not explicitly refer to spiritual aspects of health; to get agreement on this particular definition when it began in 1946, WHO drew on the input of members from many different countries that often did not agree about religion. And yet "complete physical, mental and social well-being" is really not that different from the common ideal goal of many religious traditions, though the realization of complete "spiritual" health may be defined in many different ways. The use of the word health throughout this book stands in the context of this larger discussion of an ideal that is concretely rooted in the physical body.

Public Health

"Public health" was a term created in the nineteenth century, when it was meant to refer to government-funded action related to health within a nation ("the public"). The phrase is used in a number of different ways today, but I find three descriptions particularly helpful. One is a classic definition from 1923 by Charles-Edward Amory Winslow, a founding leader in the Yale School of Public Health. It is worth giving here in full because it outlines ideas that continue to be central in global and community-based policies and practices. In this view public health is:

> The science and the art of preventing disease, prolonging life, and promoting physical health and mental health and efficiency through organized community efforts toward a sanitary environment; the control of community infections; the education of the individual in principles of personal hygiene; the organization of medical and nursing services for the early diagnosis and treatment of disease; and the development of the social machinery to ensure to every individual in the community a standard of living adequate for the maintenance of health.[19]

Another way to define the focus of public health, taken from a history written in the 1990s, goes like this:

> how populations experience health and illness, how social, economic, and political systems structure the possibilities for healthy or unhealthy lives, how societies create the preconditions for the production and transmission of disease, and how people, both as individuals and as social groups, attempt to promote their own health or avoid illness.[20]

Or, if you want a definition that is neatly short, an emergency medicine physician I know once put it like this: "disease effects within a population as they inform public policy and programming."[21]

While the common definitions of "public health" are generally distinct from those of "global health" (discussed further below), both ideas focus on what is good for whole populations—whether within or across national boundaries. Both also generally focus on action-based responses by organizations—whether governmental or those of development agencies or non-governmental organizations (NGOs, including religious NGOs)—rather than responses by individuals acting alone or in small-scale philanthropy.

Social Determinants of Health

Culture shapes who we are, including the choices we make that affect our health. We don't always have control over these cultural factors. For example, we may be at risk of lung cancer if we grew up in a household where all the adults smoked, or obesity or asthma if we grew up in the inner city where simply going outside was dangerous but the air (and lack of regular physical activity) inside our tenement was equally unhealthy. In the way we breathe, eat, move through life, and interact with substances and with other people, our encounters literally shape and change the cells in our bodies. Social circumstances that directly affect health factors are called social determinants of health. The World

Health Organization defines social determinants of health as "the circumstances in which people are born, grow up, live, work, and age, and the systems put in place to deal with illness. These circumstances are in turn shaped by a wider set of forces: economics, social policies, and politics."[22]

In fact, this idea has been around for thousands of years. Doctors, traditional healers, and religious leaders active in social reform from antiquity to the present have often prescribed relational, social, or environmental change to try to heal their patients' complaints. The modern idea as it is currently expressed took shape through concerns related to the work of the World Health Organization and political shifts that undermined or overlooked the 1978 Alma-Ata Declaration on Primary Health Care and a subsequent call for "Health for All." But many whose research and public practices of health care are deeply informed by concerns about social determinants look back in history, most often pointing first to the inspiration of a nineteenth-century German doctor named Rudolf Virchow. Virchow's 1848 "Report on the typhus epidemic in Upper Silesia" shocked many of his contemporaries around the world into recognizing that preventable and appalling living conditions among a poor population could directly lead to disastrous epidemic that no sane society would wish on its people.[23] Virchow famously insisted that "Medicine is a social science and politics is nothing more than medicine on a large scale."[24]

Health campaigns in North America and Western Europe since Virchow's day have been inconsistent in how they address the importance of social and political conditions on people's health. A return in the late 1990s to a concern with health inequities at the international level sparked renewed interest in research and public health recommendations related to social determinants. After Dr. Lee Jong-wook's appointment as director-general of the World Health Organization in 2003, one of his first activities was to call for a Commission on Social Determinants of Health (CSDH) that would release its report by 2008 (the thirtieth anniversary of Alma-Ata) "to carry forward the values that had informed global public health in its most visionary moments, translating them into practical action for a new era."[25] The CSDH report[26] led in turn to a broad array of follow-up publications, actions, and policy discussions that continue to shape global discussion of health policy reform to the present. While some global leaders committed to health equity remain frustrated by the limits of the 2008 report and what they see as the Commission's failure to effect substantial change, the phrase "social determinants of health" has become part of the common vocabulary of those who are working to make real improvements in health around the world.

The CSDH report and its related activities all focus on the present. But multidisciplinary health perspectives and influences also *cross time*. Religious history is particularly attuned to this connection with health language, and views on health and wholeness are tightly interwoven, as faith perspectives from the past continue to shape the present—and the future. Our personal health status—and the risks we face by living and breathing and getting up every day—depend on far more than just where we are and where we came from. They depend on how the place we came from got that way, as well as our capabilities for change and improvement. They depend on what our religious, cultural, and political ancestors believed, on what they did with those beliefs, and how those beliefs continue to shape the present. Addressing health across the world today calls for people who can see not only the factors that shape social determinants of health across time, but who can also think creatively about the past to imagine new possibilities for the present and future.

Global Health

Finally, what does "global health" mean as it is used in the book's title and throughout the stories that follow?

A much-used common phrase today, "global health" is often understood as little more than a synonym for what others identify as the academic disciplines of "public health" or "international health." In many schools and centers, "global health" has become a new disciplinary field within the health sciences. It is sometimes marked by turf wars over academic identity and by polite collegial distinctions to differentiate it from these two other disciplinary labels. Some critics dismiss the phrase "global health" as little more than the latest "buzz word,"[27] a concept with fuzzy boundaries that desperately needs more precise definition. As one recent editorial from the public health literature put it, "the term 'global health' does not adequately convey the real need for public health prevention and solution-oriented international work."[28]

As noted above, the word "public" in health-related discussions refers to health as it is shaped by and within a specific population. Public health usually explicitly targets government-funded or public policy-based responses, while "international" typically refers to a setting or country that is "out there," something "other" in contrast to whatever we consider to be our own home base or native culture.

For those who find themselves working in academic departments, centers, institutes, or related organizations that carry the name "global health," the phrase generally implies something broader and slightly but often distinctly different from either "public" or "international" health, supporting collaborations that are rooted in all three ideas across a range of nuances and diverse disciplines. In the perspectives that have shaped my own views most profoundly as they influenced ideas in this book, "global" looks above, beyond, and across the imposed limitations of national and continental borders to focus on the interrelated health of *everyone*, wherever they live and whatever their economic status.[29] It is about health *globally*, that is, not just in "other countries" but encompassing a concept that embraces together all countries and regions, including our own backyard. This broad view matters because it reflects how real health risks, challenges, and opportunities in today's world actually influence and shape everyone who lives in it. "Global health" is, in other words, a concept that flows: diseases, problems, and inequities that affect them cannot be fenced in; they do not stop at neighborhood or national borders. To work toward health for all, it is necessary to step outside of parochial national lenses, with their often prismatic biases about the "other," and instead to truly think like a global citizen. A global health perspective must encompass considerations of both poverty and wealth, the community and the individual body within it, and the environmental impacts of social beliefs, social actions, and social change. It is this broad meaning that informs my use of the phrase "global health" in this book, even though my particular focus is limited to looking at the role and response of religion in health disparities, and specifically, how religion impacts global health and human rights relevant to the "poor" as they face disparities that are due to the injustices of social, economic, and political inequities.

While there are many ways to illustrate what I mean by global health in this book, readers may find useful a graphic image by Dr. Kayvan Bozorgmehr, a physician who teaches social medicine, epidemiology, and health economics in Heidelberg, Germany.

This image, reproduced here (see Figure 1.1), illustrates how global health as a concept includes conditions and resources that can shape (and invite) action across three territorial dimensions. Global health has holistic meaning, says Bozorgmehr, as something that simultaneously (1) is worldwide or universal (that is, relevant in the local context of any "territory," whether town, community, country, or region across the world), (2) transcends national boundaries, and (3) relates to supraterritorial influences such as the global environment, global markets, global governance (including global governance for health), and cross-cultural interaction.

For example, a person who is coughing with a multi-drug-resistant strain of tuberculosis (MDR-TB) in, say, southern Malaysia, affects me in North America because, even in today's world, TB can be a fatal and debilitating disease regardless of modern medicine and technology; you are at risk if the drugs to

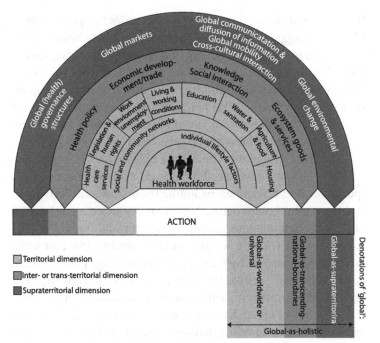

FIGURE 1.1 Global health depends on multidisciplinary intersections that cross and transcend boundaries. Graphic conceptualization from Kayvan Bozorgmehr, "Rethinking the 'Global' in Global Health: A Dialectical Approach," *Globalization and Health* 2010; 6:19, Figure 1; doi: 10.1186/1744-8603-6-19. Open access image reprinted under the terms of the Creative Commons Attribution License, (http://creativecommons. org/licenses/by/2.0), which permits unrestricted use, distribution, and reproduction in any medium, provided the original work is properly cited.

treat and cure the particular strain that you catch do not (yet) exist, if you are treated with drugs that do not work properly, or if you develop (or catch) a drug-resistant strain and then pass the bacteria on to someone else. In turn, my habits in North America affect others far away—for example, buying and throwing away lots of small appliances when they break or bore me; wasting scarce metals or adding radioactive materials to trash and land-fill; or supporting systems that compete over "food sovereignty" (like fast food chains that market junk calories from one country to another), aggravating diseases like obesity and diabetes.[30] These and related practices affect the labor demands, advertising appeal, food choices, and ultimately the living conditions and health status of workers (including children) in places that serve as suppliers to the American market (and often also handle its discarded waste). To think in terms of global health calls us to be mindful of the interconnectedness of everyone's well-being, everywhere.

The cross-disciplinary potential of global health is dazzling. Global health initiatives need input from many different sectors, specialties, and disciplines, including those who work in religion and those who hold religious beliefs and/or practice faith-based "aid" and economic interventions. Medicine and "public health" efforts are not enough; we also need innovative low-cost technologies, new approaches to social networking, public policy, governance, and creative thinking about food, advertising, and agriculture. Human gifts and capabilities include the arts. There is a rich array of research on the power of art, music, and creative expression to effect healing in disease and to encourage constructive social dynamics that are good for all. Thus, global health is also about aesthetics, beauty, and fostering one another's gifts in respect for our shared humanity. In distinguishing global health from international health in light of a definition by the Institute of Medicine, public health historian, academic, and activist Anne-Emanuelle Birn and her colleagues have described global health as "health and disease patterns in terms of the interaction of global, national, and local forces, processes, and conditions in political, economic, social, and epidemiological domains."[31] A global health vision, that is, requires collaboration that may include, for example, people in business, religious studies, engineering, technology, architecture, philosophy, art, poetry, and people from other fields who are willing to listen to one another and work together.

For health to be truly global, its means have to be fair and adequate for everyone. It is here that science intersects with ethics and moral philosophy. There is broad consensus by health and policy experts that grave health inequities are "morally unacceptable." Health disparities are not caused by technicalities like biological differences, noted the authors of a recent 2014 report of *The Lancet*—University of Oslo Commission on Global Governance for Health. Rather, they are caused by conflicting interests and power asymmetries that the authors identify as "tied to fairness and justice." Solutions require people from many different fields and walks of life to work together on these issues: "Health equity should be a cross-sectoral political concern, since the health sector cannot address these challenges alone."[32] Religion belongs in this cross-sectoral conversation about global health equity and disparities—and not just as a personal or community relationship that influences beliefs and actions about moral choice, but also and even emphatically especially as an intellectual and academic discipline.

BEHOLDEN: WHO AND TO WHOM?

The themes explored throughout this book share a single concept that is best expressed by the archaic English word, "beholden," an adjective that means "under an obligation (to), indebted" or "duty-bound."[33] The word has its roots in the Old English *behealden*, which meant "to hold, take care of, take heed, attend to, look, behold,"[34] and it evolved into *beholden* in Late Middle English. As it is used today, the word is most commonly associated with an often unwelcome sense of obligation as in, "I won't be beholden to anybody!"

Like the controversies over religious responses to global poverty, there is something discomfiting about the concept of forced obligation to another person. To "be beholden to" someone suggests that one has had a not entirely voluntary experience of being the object of another's help or beneficence, whether through some well-intentioned deed, gift-giving of some sort, or a more intangible "grace" or favor, and that this action carries with it the social and/or moral expectation that there should be some kind of payback. It implies that an exchange has taken place that now calls for one to admit and act on a debt. While the idea may include financial assistance, to "be beholden" is generally far more complicated than simple market economics. And though we may associate it with something we try to avoid, the concept of social obligation is not always seen as a bad thing. While the exchange may be called charity, philanthropy, or patronage, it is also sometimes identified using terms such as love, neighborliness, and the duties of a citizen, as well as culturally normative gift exchange. Anthropologist Mary Douglas argues (discussed further in Chapter 6) that there are "no free gifts" and that in most charitable donations "the recipient does not like the giver, however cheerful he be." Indeed, the uncomfortable global reality—assumed by religions, philosophies, and social dynamics in virtually all cultures—is that we are all beholden to one another. This book explores what that means at the intersection of religion, health, and human rights as they relate to basic economic and social needs.

TOWARD A VISION OF THE OUGHT

The idea of beholden-ness should not drag us down. Even in the Western ideal of a democratic and largely autonomous society, both health practices and human rights inevitably require social exchange, and the moral ethics of that exchange will depend on how persons treat one another. Recognizing that life in any society is to some extent about being "beholden" invites us, I suggest, into a new way of careful critical thinking about the creative dynamics of interdependence, or what historian Ted Campbell called a "vision of the ought." Writing about John Wesley's commitment to social action as an essential part of his religious beliefs, Campbell noted how "To understand a culture involves understanding a people's hopes and aspirations, understanding their vision of the ought, as well as their concept of what is. We live not only by our understanding of reality, but also by our dreams of what reality may become."[35]

This book explores how "beholden-ness" might in fact shape a vision for what is possible at the intersection of religion and global health. It is a vision for honesty about the possibilities for this intersection to cause unintended harm, but also a vision for new possibilities in interdisciplinary intersections for health strengthening. The book focuses especially on social connections within civic space, and among people who do in fact (at least sometimes) find a certain pleasure in giving—and receiving—gifts, whether they are called charity, assets, *darśan*, liturgy or worship, the affirmation of human rights, or civic justice. To explore alternative visions "of the ought" that recognize and respect the voices of religion, human rights, and health may enable new images into hope and imagination for life and health for all.

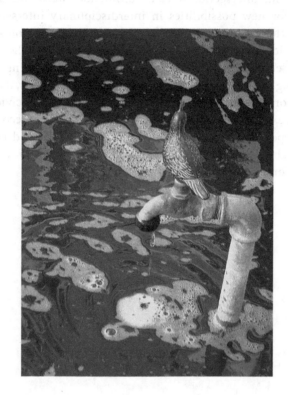

PILGRIMAGE

From "Glocality" to Global Health

"BEFORE 2001, I was a complete atheist," the seminary student told me. He and I were talking over lunch in a noisy tent in Allahabad, India, seven thousand miles from the divinity school where I had once studied early Christian cultures and he was now studying contemporary Hinduism. Across the road outside our dining tent, just beyond a small local temple, a canvas canopy shaded a gathering spot where we could gaze down from the high bluff that overlooked a floodplain, where tradition held that three sacred rivers came together in a holy space. Below the bluff, for miles across the sands, a bright patchwork of festival tents flashed and crawled with pilgrims, tourists, security police, naked and orange-clad hashish-smoking religious "sadhus," government officials, and sanitation workers. It was January in the winter of 2013, and we were at the Kumbh Mela, a sacred Hindu bathing festival that takes place in a temporary city humming and buzzing with nonstop noise from three o'clock in the morning until eleven o'clock at night. The Kumbh Mela is said to be the largest mass gathering on earth; officials estimated that in 2013 up to a hundred million people would visit this small, fifty-square-mile patch of dried-out riverbed during the fifty-five-day festival, with thirty million converging on one day alone, the most auspicious bathing day in February.[1] Far below the bluff that marked our luxury tent accommodations (complete with space heaters for the cold nights, semi-regular electricity, Western-style toilets and scheduled hot water), down along the sandbag-reinforced beach, poor villagers from across the continent mingled freely with begging children and camera-clad journalists from around the world. The event was faith in motion, shaped by the meeting point of the rivers, chief among them the Ganges, or "Mother Ganga," with her promise of purification and spiritual release to all who immersed in her waters during this auspicious season with a pure heart. The view from the bluff was muted even at noon by the smoke of a thousand altars, and before dawn each morning the dust-filled haze shimmered in the yellow electric glare like a fog sprinkled with microscopic fireflies. The river water, as I had seen close up from the beach and the bridges, was murky with the detritus of human, animal, and vegetable waste. My lunch companion's measured calm in our dining tent at the top of the bluff was a sharp contrast to the scene on the sands below.

"What happened to you in 2001?" I asked.

It was not the falling towers of Manhattan that changed his life, but an earthquake in the Indian state of Gujarat, one that registered 7.9 on the Richter scale. A former software engineer, he had been working for a nonprofit as a photojournalist. He was assigned to cover the earthquake where it had hit hardest, in a city several hours from his family's home. It was his first real journey into the face of human loss.

He would later remember a newspaper headline that appeared the following day. "Sometimes God has to show you who's boss." It was just how he felt.

Arriving at the ruined city with his camera equipment, he found a scene marked by miles of rubble. But far worse than the structural damage was the human carnage. "I began to see dead bodies," he told me. "I had never seen death before. I had only heard of people dying. And my job was to film it."

Time stood still as he walked through the wreckage. He came upon a flattened pile of shattered bricks and mortar that had been a five-story building. He could hear people underneath calling out for help. The local police began a rescue attempt, and he stayed with the diggers, filming, while trying to absorb his own internal sense of shock.

Out of the ruins diggers pulled the body of a woman, dressed, bejeweled—and decapitated. Onlookers crowded around to stare. The police asked if anyone knew her. But no one could identify her, not when they saw her as just a dead woman. However, when rescue workers began, under police supervision, to remove her jewelry and personal effects for safekeeping for the family who might claim her body, suddenly people from the crowd, realizing what she was worth, began to insist, "She was my wife" or "She was my mother." Disgusted by their greed, he turned away, heading deeper into the ruined town.

He told me how he had wandered on through the debris, still dazed. At another flattened house, he met an old man, sitting alone on steps now leading into a pile of jumbled bricks.

"'Babu,' I asked—for this is how we address old men with respect—'Are you alright? Have you lost anyone?' And he looked up at me and laughed. 'I have lost my entire family,' he said. 'My three sons. My three daughters-in-law. My grandchildren. My wife. They are lying—right here.' And he pointed down at the ruins where he sat.

"What could I say?" the student wondered aloud. "I offered him some tea that I had with me. I was overwhelmed for him. But he smiled at me.

"'Why are you upset?' the old man asked. 'Do you not know the Hindu scriptures? We are born. We die. We are born again. I am 75 years old. I have maybe four or five years left until I die. If they had lived and I had died, they would grieve for me. Now they will not grieve. Why grieve, when this is what we are told happens to every person?'" And he again smiled at the young journalist, both chiding and comforting.

"And then," the student told me, "he recited something. It was from the Hindi scriptures, a saying that my mother used to recite to us at night when we were children. It had never meant anything to me before. But now—recited by this old man in this terrible place—I understood it for the first time." In that moment something happened, and religion took on a new meaning, a new truth and value for him.

The old man asked what he would do, and if he would help other people. "Yes," he told him, "I will do my work as I must—but I will also spend a portion of my time to help others." And the old man asked him, "Can I come with you?"

"He stayed with me for several weeks," the student told me. "He became like my family. I told him, 'You are like my father and I am your son.'" Transformed by this religious experience, the student would eventually find his way to graduate school, not to advance his career in software engineering or the media, but as a divinity school student seeking further understanding in the diversities and depth of faith in action, practical faith in a personal commitment to justice, and to peace.

THE "GLOCALITY" OF GLOBAL HEALTH

The student's story that day at lunch moved me deeply. It was not just because I knew his reputation as a gentle and committed religious activist for peace and justice. It was also because I too understood, on a personal level, the distinction between religious faith and the academic study of religion. Reflective academic research—which had brought us both to the Kumbh Mela—is vital for understanding how health, social justice, and religion can work together, but such intellectual understanding is only a part of what it can mean to take faith-based issues seriously. Indeed, I was living that week in a particular tension between these two very different worlds. On one hand, I was there to think creatively about the academic study of global health, as part of a cross-university project to explore the multidisciplinary relationships among religion, business, urban design, environmental issues, public health, and clinical medicine as they affected aspects of wellness across cultures and lives. But on the other hand, our collective and open-air "classroom" at the festival had validity and meaning only in the context of the living faith that the pilgrims and religious teachers around us sought to integrate into the whole person in a life-changing encounter. While I had come to India as an academic, the student's story over lunch pushed me back into reflections that dissolved my neat intellectual boxes with the force of the ever-present truth that piety is personal. And because it is personal, its effects on humanitarian relief and social justice often shape the impulses of our heart and take us by surprise. Such surprise is sometimes sharpest when we are forced out of our comfort zones, when global and local elide. As South African theologian Steve de Gruchy and colleagues once put it, "We live in a context of 'glocality': our local lives are affected by global processes."[2]

We do not need to travel to another country to learn this. The student, for example, had found it in 2001 just a few hours away from his home. In its "dance" between faith-based responses to human need and the role of religion in contemporary health issues, the personal impact of such glocality lives in the multifaceted vortex of global health as a cross-disciplinary and multidimensional concept on our own skin, in our encounters with what we see, think, feel, and do, in relationship to one another. This is in itself a sort of pilgrimage, a sacred journey to new lessons in life, and perhaps also a form of migration, a discomforting transition to a shift in one's encounter with life itself.

During the rest of my time in India that week, I continued to think about the student's story, the "glocality" of pilgrimage, and its role in global health across the centuries. My thoughts were further shaped by the very physical world I was encountering through the enforced pilgrimage and temporary "migration" of my own journey to the Kumbh. Although I was not a Hindu, I too was there to learn from the festival, and the only way to do that had been to travel and experience it firsthand. Even an admittedly academic pilgrimage nonetheless shapes the traveler through the immediacy of group life in such a journey—its impact on one's flesh and bones. For those of us at the Kumbh Mela, this meant the impact of life in a tent, the health risks of food, water, travel, insects, and contagion, and interpersonal dynamics with another culture, language, noise level, and crowd density.

Our own group context at the Kumbh—and the range of pilgrims we encountered during the trip—was easily as diverse as that wonderful medley of characters in the most classic pilgrimage account of all, Chaucer's *Canterbury Tales*. When lunch ended that Sunday afternoon, and the student left our table to join a group that would gather at the sacred beach area known as the *sangam*, I stayed in the dining tent a little longer, making notes and watching my fellow travelers.

It was a curious study in contrasts. At that moment, for example, moving shadows in the tent doorway heralded the entrance of another student, one accompanied by his new guru—a tall dreadlock-and-orange-cotton-clad *sadhu* from the fair. Both of them were smiling beatifically. Behind him, our camp manager followed, serious and clearly distracted. He was a biology professor's son from Goa, a Roman Catholic, who had opted out of graduate school for a career in four-star hospitality. Now he was turning to welcome into the tent a group very different from the half-naked Hindu teachers that dominated the festival: a staid and neatly dressed Catholic priest accompanied by nine or ten Indian Catholic nuns, all in full habit. Others in the tent turned to stare. I had attended the priest's church that morning, and knew that he directed a nearby Catholic hospital, where the camp director had brought several guests a few days earlier for emergency medical care. Across the room at another table, three American emergency medicine physicians from Boston, a Caucasian Episcopalian and two doctors of South Asian ethnicity, were discussing logistics for a health-based project to combine a "cloud" technology for medical records with the challenge of moving volunteer doctors fast through the dense crowds of pilgrims attending the *sangam* and the festival's ten sector clinics. At the table beside the doctors, graduate students in architectural design were poised over an exquisitely drawn map, comparing it with their laptop details of the festival's city plan. In another corner, a veteran public health expert, Dr. Richard Cash, renowned for his work on treating cholera, was chatting about infectious diseases with two public health graduate students, a pharmacist and a dentist. On the path outside, I could see business school students hurrying to talk with vendors in the local markets. And one of our co-leaders, religious studies professor Diana Eck, was with her students at that moment out on the beach with several Hindu NGOs in a collaborative faith-based river cleanup exercise as part of a "Green Kumbh" movement, one that would be broadcast around the world on television that evening. Her work gave voice to the living religion—lived theology—that connected these many dots between ideas of wellness and urban design that defined our group's purpose at the festival. It is these related and overlapping strands, I thought as I got up to leave, that global health is all about: a constructive intersection that crosses disciplinary and community sectors and gains its very strength from the diversities.

"But what am I doing here?" This was a question I asked myself silently and often that week despite the clarity of our group's collaborative purposes. My religious tradition of Christianity, and my personal expressions of it, are in many ways radically different from Hinduism, even as I appreciate ecumenical dialogue and those immutable distinctions that shape the real boundaries and points of differences that demand respect within and across faith communities. As I prepared for the trip, from visa applications to immunizations, I found myself wondering, "How can I honestly wrap my mind—my whole self and all that shapes who I am and how I think—around this religious and yet profoundly alien event?"

Trying to make sense of the Kumbh Mela—and my personal presence in the midst of it—I found it helpful to look back at the history of Christian pilgrimage, something I knew about, together with its rich traditions rooted in a similar journey toward health.

PILGRIMAGE, POVERTY, AND SOCIAL JUSTICE: SEEKING HEALTH ACROSS TIME

Pilgrimage is a journey to and into the holy. Most pilgrims to the Kumbh Mela, it is said, are poor villagers, but they come not because they are poor, but because they are human persons of faith (see Figure 2.1). As I walked along the roads at the festival, crossed the metal-plate pontoon bridges, and stood on straw-covered sandbags at the touchpoint of the rivers' confluence,

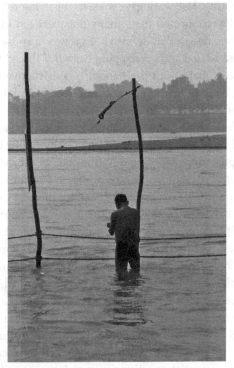

FIGURE 2.1 Pilgrim at the Kumbh Mela festival performs a sacred bathing ritual in the Ganges River at Allahabad, India. Author photo.

surrounded by a rainbow of wet cloth, begging children, unpredictable and pious travelers of all ages, I thought about how social justice and global health issues intersect with pilgrimage stories across history. Something I had read about comparative theology before the trip was especially helpful, a quote from an essay by Francis X. Clooney, a Jesuit who has spent his life in dialogue with Hinduism and who knows well the creative tensions of inter-religious discussion. Clooney has defined comparative theology as "learning across religious borders in a way that discloses the truth of my faith, in the light of their faith."[3] Distinct from personal faith, comparative theology is "not primarily about which religion is the true one,"[4] he says, but rather an open, honest, and detached learning process: "about God, whose grace keeps making room for all of us as we find our way faithfully in a world of religious diversity."[5] In both Hindu and early Christian traditions, the pilgrimage community crosses literal as well as physical (and sometimes even shared religious) boundaries in expectation of some holistic gain or blessing.[6] Social justice and even equity are common threads in many pilgrimage stories.

Consider, for example, Simeon the Stylite. Perched atop a sixty-foot pillar for forty years in fifth-century Edessa in Syria, Simeon practiced public prayer as he also dispensed food, medicine, and justice. Each afternoon, he taught and heard disputes, "sitting in judgment and handing down proper and just sentences." His views on money-lending resonate with twenty-first-century "Jubilee" movements, debt justice, and forgiveness activism, as he called for radical reform, reducing loan interest to one half percent per month (6 percent per year) and often urging people to forgive the interest entirely.[7] As Syriac scholar Susan Ashbrook Harvey has noted, "Simeon's body bore the truth of the world he saw: the suffering, the terror, the weariness, and the radiance of transfigured grace."[8]

The Kumbh Mela at Allahabad may also have historical links with other instances of pillar climbing. A seventh-century Chinese travel narrative by a Buddhist monk, Huien Tsang, described ascetic "heretics" (meaning non-Buddhists) whom he observed climbing pillars in the Ganges River in ancient Prayag—modern Allahabad, indeed at the site of today's Kumbh Mela.[9] Huien Tsang had gone to India looking for manuscripts, and some consider his travelogue to be one of the first references to an early version of the Kumbh Mela. In the middle of the river, he said, "dozens" of ascetics climbed a column each day at sunset, hanging their bodies out over the river while holding on with one hand and foot, gazing into the setting sun. Their hope, he noted, was "to escape from birth and death." They followed this practice, Huien Tsang noted, daily for decades.

Huien Tsang described another event on the sand between the rivers—that flat plain that was crowded in 2013 with tents, pilgrims, hashish-smoking ascetics, and reporters with video cameras. For Huien Tsang, this area was called the "great charity enclosure." Here, he said, the rich and noble gathered, "whenever they had occasion to distribute their gifts in charity." According to his account, the local king would lead off in something that sounds like what anthropologists call a "potlatch" divestment, that is, one of extravagant mutual gifting that effectively impoverishes the donor. These began with donations to a statue of Buddha, followed by distributions according to descending social rank: to the priests, leaders, non-Buddhists, and lastly to the widows and bereaved, orphans and desolate, poor and mendicants. Once the poor had bowed and scraped from the bottom of the barrel, the king would cry out with joy, "Well done! Now all that I have has entered into incorruptible and imperishable treasuries!" (If this sounds a bit like the New Testament, it may be because Samuel Beal, who translated the Chinese text into English, had been a British chaplain in Queen Victoria's Royal Navy.) But if we expect the Indian king to make a radical conversion to asceticism like St. Antony of Egypt or Simeon of the Syrian desert, we are in for a surprise. For after this radical divestment, Huien Tsang says, "the rulers of the different countries offer their jewels and robes to the king, so that his treasury is replenished." The divestment is linked, here, that is, to a domino-like exchange of giving that ends with a restoration of the preexisting social order.

Such profligate gift exchange seems somewhat distant from poverty relief or justice, even if the poor play a bit part. The cycle that Huien Tsang describes may indeed have been shaped most profoundly by the ascetic value of Buddhist detachment. And yet the large-scale local investment in a public display and religious exchange does curiously match the underlying theological spirit of the modern Hindu Kumbh Mela. Pilgrim encounters with the ascetic sadhus—traditionally fierce warriors who are even today the real power behind the religious event—continue to include lavish gift exchange. The ascetics give money and food to the pilgrims, who, in turn, give gifts (including money) back to the holy person in respect, gratitude, and exchange for the blessing of something called *darśan*, which Diana Eck defines as "auspicious sight." This holy gaze in Hinduism, she says, involves looking at not only temple places and shrines but also visual engagement with living teachers, ascetics, and sadhus who are believed to embody the holy: "Beholding the image is an act of worship, and through the eyes one gains the blessings of the divine."[10] While darśan is something specific to Hinduism, historians of Christianity have also emphasized the importance of the sacred "gaze" in both modern religious art and late antique travelogues about holy healing.[11]

As the exchange that Huien Tsang witnessed was apparently marked by both Buddhist and non-Buddhist influences, so too other ancient pilgrimage narratives hint at similar intersections that cross religious boundaries. Christian healing saints' stories from late antiquity often speak of Christian and Muslim pilgrims together revering the same sacred sites. We find this ecumenical diversity in other saints' traditions as well. Two hundred years before Huien Tsang went wandering in search of good books among the non-Buddhist "heretics" of India, Fa Hsien, another Buddhist priest exploring India in the early fifth century, described how "the elders and gentry" had instituted free hospitals that served "all poor or helpless patients, orphans, widowers, and cripples" with food, medicine, and comforting healing care.[12] Similar religious diversity is evident in a ninth-century medical handbook for pilgrims to Mecca (discussed below) which, while obviously intended for Muslim pilgrims, was written by a Christian physician who drew on earlier (including pre-Christian) Greek science and philosophy.

THE GIFT OF WATER

Pilgrims often travel to a holy site expecting to die. Similarly, travelers forced into migration by economics, war, or natural disasters often also face mortal risks that challenge both health and religious practices. At the steps that lead down into the Ganges River throughout India, for example, it is not uncommon for a traveler or tourist to be invited (or forced in the course of ordinary events) to view a dead body.[13] As death and water are often related facts in the transitions of both pilgrims and refugees, so too death and water may also serve as markers that tell us what life was like for those who themselves suffered health risks far from home. Imagery of water—as it relates to both purity and disease at pilgrimage sites—as well as physical markers of such migration—in bones and teeth from ancient cemeteries, for example—can tell us a great deal about the everyday life and physical transitions of both rich and poor across history. Such evidence sometimes also hints at the inequities they faced and the role of their faith in healing efforts.

Water flows through most pilgrimage and travel texts. Concerns include how to be sure you have it, whether you have enough, and what it is likely to do to your physical and spiritual constitution. At the Kumbh Mela, for example, pilgrims come to have their sins washed away by "Mother Ganga," and yet one sees here none of the certainty common to baptism in Protestant Christianity—that "one dip does it all." Bathing at the *sangam*—that most holy spot of water where the sacred Ganges, Yamuna, and (historical but now legendary) Saraswati rivers meet—is a repetitive act, with many pilgrims returning every morning of their stay, and many coming back again at subsequent festivals. While pilgrims come seeking release from the endless cycle of reincarnation and the assurance of a blissful death, fatalities are something that the Kumbh Mela officials and health providers prefer to avoid and prevent. Indeed, officials' greatest concern over the decades has been to minimize the risk of accidents and water-borne disease, particularly cholera. These fears are not unwarranted; several cholera epidemics have been associated with the festival, and some epidemiologists and medical historians even suggest that the 1817 Kumbh Mela was possibly responsible for triggering the worldwide cholera pandemic in the nineteenth century.[14]

The salvific nature of water at pilgrimage sites and pre-Christian sanctuaries—such as those of Asclepius in ancient Greece associated with sacred springs—was also an important aspect of many martyr sanctuaries and pilgrimage sites in late antiquity. In fourth-century Cappadocia, for example, pilgrims flocked to the church and shrine of St. Julitta, a martyr whose voluntary death on a Roman sacrificial pyre, according to hagiography, transformed the very ground into a healing spring.[15] And near what was perhaps the location of Basil of Caesarea's fourth-century hospital complex for the poor, one of the most renowned hospitals in early Christian history and said to have been located "a little outside the city [walls],"[16] there stands today in modern Kayseri an early thirteenth-century Islamic structure known as the "Gevher Nesibe" complex. While it is not associated (as far as I know) with any ancient Roman Christian remains, this complex too was once a hospital, religious space, and training setting for medical students that included bathing facilities.[17] Such places are reminders that health concerns—and legendary philanthropic founders of free health care for the poor—continue to shape history and politics across religious borders and across time.

As seventh-century pilgrims in India were hanging from pillars in the Ganges, Christians in Egypt appealed to God for physical healing and spiritual cleansing through holy doctors—saints like the Evangelist Luke as well as martyr-saints like Cyrus and John, Cosmas and Damian, and others, sometimes called *anargyroi*, or doctors who healed for free. Others combined faith with practical medical care as part of their living support for the local community; we see this, for example, in the lives of bishops like Rabbula of Edessa[18] in sixth-century Syria or John the Almsgiver[19] in early seventh-century Egypt.[20] In both healing shrines and hospitals, the sick body was likely to receive therapy that included food, drink, bathing, worship, and often bizarre or startling treatments that force the patient into the saint's view of right moral relationship with the holy and one another. While medicinal springs in eighteenth- and nineteenth-century Europe and North America would come to be valued independent of particular religious beliefs, their cultural and medical claims continued to illustrate the value of water in philosophical perspectives on health. Dr. William Trevitt, for example—whose story is told in the next chapter—was fascinated by the role of water in treating cholera and other diseases, and his report on the purported medicinal effects of the mineral waters of Ohio, published in the *Ohio Medical and Surgical Journal* in March 1857, speaks to an era in which the rich might spend their holidays "taking the water" at some celebrated spa.

BUT IS THE WATER CLEAN?

When Brandeis University professor Joseph Lumbard was studying Arabic as a young American convert to Islam, he spent one of his last evenings in Morocco enjoying a quiet visit to the courtyard of an ancient mosque in the city of Fez. There he met an old man who was serving water to those in the courtyard. When the old man learned that Lumbard had embraced Islam as an adult as a result of personal choice, the man "began to cry, got down on his knees, hugged me, and kissed me," Lumbard recalls, and then filled a cup from his bucket and presented it to him as a gift "in the name of Allah." Pondering the proffered cup, Lumbard wrote,

> I knew I would get sick, but I also felt I had to accept. And indeed, the generosity and hospitality of this old man was something that I quite literally carried home with me, unfortunately in the form of giardia. Nonetheless this has always been one of my most cherished memories. For in his instant of joy that man felt he had to do something to offer hospitality to the stranger. With nothing on him and probably with few possessions other than the bare necessities, there was only one thing, a cup of water. Yet at the same time, I had learned something . . . that I often forget elsewhere, namely, that hospitality is a two-way street.[21]

Water is about as basic as health and gift can get. It is easy to forget that water is not just a precious resource, but also in fact an essential nutrient for health. The Institute of Medicine of the National Academies of Science's Food and Nutrition Board's "Dietary Reference Intakes" (DRIs)—the national standards for basic dietary needs—reflects this reality by including recommendations for water.[22]

Both food and water are—at least in theory—recognized as international rights.[23] In 2002, the United Nations Committee on ESC Rights (CESCR) adopted General Comment 15 on the Right to Water, finding that "the human right to safe drinking water and sanitation" is contained within the right to an adequate standard of living and thus relates to the right to health in the International Covenant on ESC Rights (ICESCR, discussed further in Chapter 4). In 2010, the UN adopted resolutions that further affirm the existence of a right to safe drinking water and sanitation. Applying this right to law, however, remains complex.[24]

Water is tragically easy to waste and pollute. Preventable diarrheal fluid loss from water-borne infections, often related to malnutrition, is one of the primary reasons infants die around the world today. Toxic waste from industrial pollution—mercury or chromium, for example—are also known pollutants in water that can have fatal or debilitating effects that cannot be boiled away, with often gruesome consequences for their victims. Making water a global "gift" for health may call for acts as simple as teaching children to control faucet flow to avoid waste, or changing cross-border policies and innovative low-cost technologies that control wastewater treatment and improve water purity and toilet sanitation where it counts.

The only known health guide for Muslim pilgrims to Mecca from the ancient world devotes nearly a quarter of its advice to the subject of water. Written a thousand years before the discovery of bacteria, its attention to water sanitation sounds surprisingly modern. "The best water is that which is tasteless, odourless and colourless," wrote the author, a Christian doctor named Qusṭā ibn Lūqā al-Baʿlabakkī (ca. 820–912 CE).[25] If one must drink "contaminated" water (which he describes as water that has any taste, color, or smell, including water from snow or ice and water "collected in places hidden from the sun"[26]), Qusṭā says, boil it well first, and he emphasizes, "I mean on a fire." And if it is not clear, he adds, then strain it several times. The author of this treatise was a scholar and linguist from Syria who served under several Muslim rulers, in Baghdad and in Armenia, translating Greek science into Arabic. Qusṭā wrote his treatise to be a practical guide when his family responsibilities ("my dear young children who cannot be left alone"[27]) prevented him from accompanying his patron on the pilgrimage to Mecca. Although Christians usually were not allowed in Mecca, accompanying physicians were the occasional exception.

In another pilgrimage text, William Wey, a fifteenth-century English priest (and possible spy for the king) also includes comments on staying healthy in his 1458 pilgrimage account of travels

to Rome, Venice, Jaffa, and Jerusalem. Wey particularly emphasizes the importance of traveling with a 10-gallon barrel of water
and including in the travel contract that the ship's *patron* promises "that the wine that you will drink shall be good and your
water fresh, provided that it is obtainable."[28]

LEARNING FROM BONES

Like disease, poverty—as well as pilgrimage, whether chosen
or forced—can also leave its mark on the body. Social determinants of health (defined in Chapter 1) that suggest economic destitution are often evident in data from research that
examines health factors through the lens of culture, archaeology, and material evidence of religious practices in the distant
past. Anthropologist Tracy L. Prowse, for example, has used
data from carbon and nitrogen isotopes and dental evidence
to examine the health of people in what was probably a workers' graveyard on an imperial Roman estate.[29] One third of the
people she studied were young children. Among the adults, she
found evidence that the men's diet was likely higher in pro-
tein than that of the women. She also found gender differences
in the bone evidence of healed fractures, with men breaking
bones in their lower limbs and women more often in the chest
and upper limbs.[30] These differences imply varying patterns of
stressful activities related to lifestyle and work. Men's teeth had
significantly more cavities than women's, also suggesting they
had a better diet with more frequent food.[31]

Luigi Capasso, a physician who has worked on the human
remains from Pompeii and Herculaneum, has also identified
dietary and health factors in this ancient Roman population.
Evidence of chronic lung infections, for example, suggested indoor
air pollution from the carbon by-products of burning lamps and
cookfires.[32] Capasso also noted work-related bone lesions called
syndesmoses, which occurred only on one side of the body, found

for example in the bones of one eight-year-old child,[33] suggesting heavy manual labor, perhaps from farming or rowing the single-oar Roman boats.[34]

Archaeologist and religious historian Leonard Rutgers has likewise been able to document health conditions for skeletons found in 3,700 graves in the Roman catacombs, even specifying them according to age, gender, and bone growth (or stunting as a result of chronic malnutrition).[35] Other scholars have identified the effects of slavery[36] or evidence of damage caused by ascetic religious practices, such as repetitive liturgical kneeling, in monastic skeletons.[37] Similar studies from different historical periods have looked at the effects of other aspects of religious practice on the human body of those who may not have shared the faith convictions that caused their unhealthy behaviors. Archaeologist Barry Kemp's recent study on the workers' cemetery at Egyptian Pharaoh Akhenaton's sacred city of Tell el Amarna, for example, provides a startling clinical exposé of how this "heretic" king's religious zeal created fatally abusive working conditions for thousands of ordinary peasants.[38]

CONCLUSION

It has been said that "visits to the other can result in the confluence of images that will never be erased from memory . . . too complex for neat and rigid categorization."[39] Such transitional journeying, whether one is visiting a culture next door or across the world, is also an essential aspect of global health, particularly as it relates to religion. It was certainly my experience at the Kumbh Mela, and, on a deeper level, also the experience of the student who encountered the slaughter of natural disaster in the Gujarat earthquake. Whether contemporary clinical reports or archaeological evidence from a body in ancient history, such evidence helps to illustrate how global health, issues of rights and entitlements, and faith-based actions toward global economic and social justice are not primarily about international aid, but rather part of everyday life. They take place in the activities that make us human and keep us in motion: worship, travel, work, migration, the quest for health, and encounters with disease and death. A faith-based perspective with a global health lens calls for a broad-scope awareness of a diversity of stories from across disciplines and communities, as we seek to live out our own story with integrity. Such narratives and places serve as reminders that the individual body, ill or healthy, is shaped—literally—by its culture as it absorbs the material world.[40]

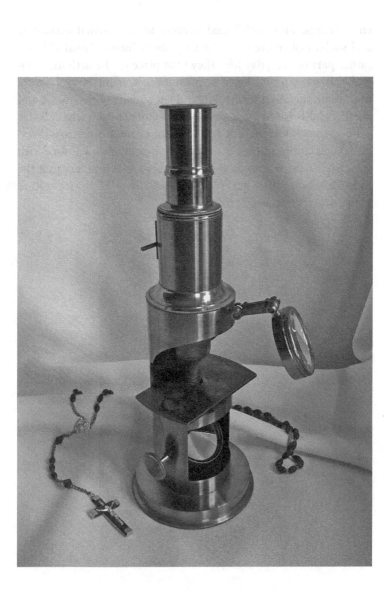

PRIVATE LENS, PUBLIC HEALTH

A Reluctant Physician in Nineteenth-Century America

"SO YOU ARE reading medicine—I am glad to hear it. You must stick to it now. Don't change your mind again."[1]

With these words Captain John Trevitt, a West Point–trained Army physician stationed in upstate New York and getting ready to join his regiment in the Republic of Texas on the Rio Grande, wrote to his twenty-three-year-old brother, Henry, in Columbus, Ohio, in May 1846. Ever the authoritarian older brother (though there were only two years between them), John was feeling out of sorts that week, waiting to see the dentist for a toothache. He was trying to be helpful. "When you come to the lectures," he added, "I will assist you if the Mexicans have not eaten me up."

John's letter to Henry was another surprise I found in my grandmother's trunk, described in Chapter 1. I had known of Dr. Henry Trevitt (see Figure 3.1) since childhood. In our family's oral traditions about the past, Henry's story consisted of a few facts, a small collection of physical objects his widow had passed on to my grandmother, and a strange silence. The little I knew touched directly on my own interests—his work in public health medicine, his service as an "overseer of the poor," and a hint that he had participated in an international encounter. I wanted to know more. What had public health medicine meant for Henry, and how was it practiced in his world? Given the importance of religion in the ethical

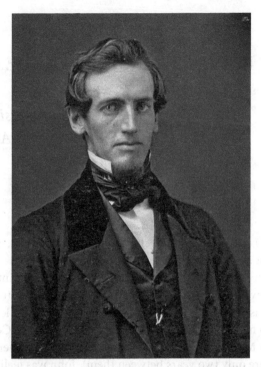

FIGURE 3.1 Henry Trevitt, ca. 1850. This daguerreotype may have been produced in his studio in downtown Columbus, Ohio. Laterally reversed to correct for the mirror image of daguerreotype photography. Photo courtesy of the author.

narratives about medicine in nineteenth-century America, where did religion shape his life choices? I knew that he had "directed" an American hospital in Chile during a year spent with his uncle on political business, but what had that year been like, I wondered, and how had it influenced the thirty years that followed, as a rural country druggist and overseer of the poor in southern New Hampshire? Were those last years really as idyllic as I had been led to believe? His brother's letter was my first hint that Henry's medical career was perhaps less than the heroic cipher of family tradition.

And what might Henry's story suggest about the role of history in shaping American health policies that continue to influence philanthropic and public health care coverage decisions in the United States today and in American interests abroad? While many of the details I would learn about him are outside the focus of this book, Henry's career in the context of the history of public health and nineteenth-century religious responses to poverty, the subject of this chapter, does indeed suggest much that is relevant to the complexity of global health today.

By the time John sent off his nuggets of brotherly advice, it had been six years since Henry had left home, at seventeen, to follow John's lead as a medical student—and still he had nothing to show for it. In fact, it was to be another decade, despite John's goading, before Henry would take up medicine seriously.

The pressure on Henry to study medicine must have been immense. He was the youngest of three surviving children in a family of military and medical patriots in early America. Henry was named after both his great-grandfather—who fought and died in the bloody battle of Fort William Henry in the French-American war of 1757 (popularized in the twentieth century by the movie, "The Last of the Mohicans")—and his grandfather, a Revolutionary War patriot who had emigrated to frontier Ohio at the venerable age of seventy-four in 1829, when Henry was six, and would live on into his nineties. By the 1840s, all four of Henry and John's surviving paternal uncles had followed the old man's trail to Ohio.

Henry and John were likely most influenced by the two uncles who had gone into medicine. The older uncle—also named John—was a family hero. We learn about him through the pen of Sarah Jane Trevitt, Henry and John's only surviving sister (see Figure 3.2). Born in 1818, Sarah Jane would spend her long life at home in Mont Vernon, where she gained some prominence as a landscape painter and art teacher. At age 56, after both her parents died, she got married for the first time, to another physician in the village who had recently lost his wife. Later in life she wrote

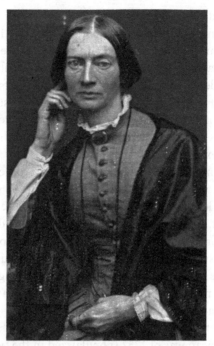

FIGURE 3.2 Sarah Jane Trevitt in the 1850s, when she was in her mid-thirties. Daguerreotype most likely taken by her brother, Henry. Laterally reversed to correct for the mirror image of daguerreotype photography. Photo courtesy of the author.

a short history of the Trevitt family for the benefit of her brothers' children, a narrative that I was to find matched the most reliable of the surviving public records with extraordinary accuracy.[2] She provides the greatest detail for the lives of those who became physicians.

The older of her two physician uncles, John Trevitt, born in 1790, began his medical studies as an apprentice with a local New Hampshire physician. This apprenticeship model was the norm, though young Henry would experience first-hand its transition into the modern focus on structured classroom and clinical training during his years at Starling Medical College in Ohio in the late 1850s. After serving in the War of 1812 as an army surgeon, uncle John had spent the next decade in adventures traveling across pioneer country, from Vermont to New York, Detroit, Michigan, and Fort Wayne, Indiana. From there, wrote Sarah Jane, he marched with the army "south to Mobile Point after a long tedious journey through the wilderness," where the troops were "ordered to East and West Florida." John's final station, his niece noted, "was Augusta Georgia and there he died in 1821 of yellow fever." Sarah Jane adds a parenthetical note on her source: "(This information was gained from letters which he sent to my father regularly from every post)." In fact (though Sarah Jane does not say so), John was part of the Seminole Wars, a campaign led by General (later President) Andrew Jackson to suppress and kill Native Americans as well as the British and Spanish troops who were believed to support the Indians during the European settlement of Georgia and Florida.[3]

The example of this pioneer physician had its most immediate influence on his youngest brother, William. Born in 1808, William was a child when John joined the army and a teenager when he died in Augusta.

William Trevitt, like his older brother John, also first apprenticed under a local village doctor in New Hampshire followed by formal studies in medicine at Dartmouth and then, in 1830, at the University of Philadelphia. From there, he emigrated West to follow his grandfather and three other brothers to Ohio, where he was soon known for his dedication at treating victims of the 1832 cholera epidemic. In 1837 his nephew John joined him; John was sixteen. Three years later, in 1840, as John went on to West Point, William was elected secretary of state, moving to Columbus. It was at this juncture that Henry "left New Hampshire," Sarah Jane wrote, "and went to Ohio to study medicine with his uncle William."

Sarah Jane says little more about the next eighteen years in Henry's life except to note that "While his uncle was Sec. of State, he was his clerk." William held this political appointment during three terms, from 1840 to 1841 and then again between 1852 and 1856. And public records do attest to Henry's role as a clerk in the State House in the mid-1850s; he was certainly not studying medicine.

Not that he lacked opportunity. William Trevitt was a zealous physician who maintained a private practice wherever he could. He was also eager to serve the public, and to benefit from pioneer real estate opportunities. He spent much of these years buying up land, investigating Ohio's natural springs, investing in the construction of public institutions such as elementary schools as well as the local insane asylum, and serving as state-appointed physician to the penitentiary.[4] When cholera struck again in 1849 and the leading prison physician died of it, William stepped in as the interim physician, soon publishing his success at reducing mortality in the weeks that followed. William was also dedicated to improving medical education, promoting classroom training and codes of accountability, and serving on several boards for the nascent Starling Medical College (later the University of Columbus Medical School), where young Henry eventually received his MD in 1860. The lives of both William and Henry offer a snapshot of a formative era in American public health, an era shaped by the spirit of pioneering adventure, patriotism, and civic and religious duty as they engaged with emerging and globalizing medical practices for poor and suffering citizens at home and abroad.

In his social history of welfare in America and the history of the American poorhouse, Michael Katz has emphasized the importance of considering the actions of private citizens in close association with public policies in the nineteenth and early twentieth centuries. "Voluntarism never was and never will be able to meet the needs of poor and dependent Americans," he wrote. "Public welfare always has supported more dependent people than private relief. In fact, it is virtually impossible to disentangle the private from the public in social welfare."[5]

This intersection between private and public was often marked and motivated during the nineteenth century by faith-based ideals that were held by ordinary citizens working within public and government systems. We saw this in Chapter 1, in Benjamin Rush's call for universal health care, the abolition of slavery, and human dignity for the poor, actions that required an intersection between public and private and which followed from deep religious beliefs. The fact that Rush's views were regarded as liberal generosity in his day highlights the contrast between his view and the conservative biases and assumptions of many of his peers. While Katz has contrasted public policy with the "private" acts of individual voluntarism, the story of the Trevitt doctors—together with examples of religious service to the poor sick in chaplain and missionary efforts across the nineteenth century—can help illustrate how private lives also profoundly shaped public activities. It is these moral and civic duties—a public sense of being "beholden" to others for the common good—that would deeply shape the background and experiences of young Henry Trevitt throughout his reluctant medical career. It was a career marked by encounters with corrupt government, revolution, mental illness, prison medicine, international scandal, and small-town murder.

PREACHING WELFARE IN NINETEENTH-CENTURY AMERICA

The American welfare system during the eighteenth and nineteenth centuries was developed broadly on the model of earlier English poor laws. These used local administration (in England the church parish) to fund public aid that would help keep the local indigent alive (if only barely) and (if they were physically capable) hard at work.[6] In nineteenth-century America such public policies focused not on the church but on the local town political and tax structure, while churches provided the moral education for citizens who might offer volunteer work or serve the community through civic public action. This church-state distinction in America throughout this period functioned synergistically, with citizens, doctors, and clergy working together to support a sense of social order and "common good." While such aid served the poor both in their own homes and in group settings, institutions were increasingly seen as the best answer to care for the needy who could not care for themselves. Often, private personal tragedies lie just below the surface of such institutional narratives. Benjamin Rush's concern for institutions for the mentally ill, for example, was likely shaped by the insanity of his oldest son, who lost his wits as an adult after training as a military surgeon and spent the rest of his life locked in an asylum.[7] One witness to this trend in institutional care for the needy, the Rev. Ezra Stiles Ely in New York City in 1810 said that "the asylum for maniacs and the orphan asylum, are monuments of praise to those who have endowed them. . . . Shall I forget to name the Almshouse, the Hospital, and the State Prison?"[8] And frontier cities like Columbus, Ohio proudly illustrated their city maps with the "notable locations," often monumental in size and elaborate architecture, of institutions such as schools for the blind or for the deaf and dumb, the penitentiary, "lunatic asylum," and county infirmary.[9]

Institutions for the sick poor were nothing new. For example, early Christian sources from the Roman empire in the fifth and sixth centuries, including laws, church rules, saints' lives, monastic descriptions, and the evidence of archaeology, all attest to the widespread construction and use of orphanages, old-age homes, and hospitals, including hospitals for lepers, strangers, insane monks, poor women in childbirth, and other targeted medical conditions.[10] Most early Christian welfare institutions were staffed by monks, nuns, and slaves—in other words, forced volunteers. The existence of such institutions, which followed a very similar model up to the Protestant

Reformation (and beyond) does not necessarily imply or prove that the people they were said to serve were treated kindly.[11] There is an abundant history of such institutional-based religious health care in other ancient religious traditions. When the Protestant Reformation destroyed the funding base of many monastic facilities, leading to their collapse and closure, some reformers in Europe, like Ulrich Zwingli and John Calvin, were to shape entire new civic legal systems based on alternative ways to aid the indigent sick in their midst, restructuring but essentially maintaining institutional models.[12] Some of these civic models shaped Puritan systems in colonial America. By the nineteenth century, public health policies engaged both this historical value for religious charity to an organized group and a "secular" value for moral duty as a responsible citizen.

William Trevitt was a toddler and his brother John was serving as a medical apprentice when Ezra Stiles Ely, a Presbyterian clergyman, spent the year preaching to drunks, beggars, and prostitutes in the City Hospital and Almshouse in New York City. As part of an appeal for funding, Ely published a tract titled *A Sermon for the Rich to Buy that They May Benefit Themselves and the Poor.*[13] The tract targeted potential donors, including those with government influence, calling for the creation of an endowment that could be used to fund hospital chaplains like himself. Hospitals at this time were principally bleak open halls or homes for the poor who lacked family or any means of private medical care. The importance of sanitation for health and medical care was unknown, and public hospital facilities often crowded the sick together in a manner that surely helped to spread communicable diseases. Ely's appeal called for the reader to give up a few small personal pleasures in order to invest in the poor:

> Tax your luxuries . . . forsake the theatre, and abstain from the
> fourth glass of wine throughout the year, and a fund would
> soon be raised, the interest of which should supply a chaplain

with the necessaries of life, who should visit the destitute sick, and preach three or four discourses weekly, to such as are ready to perish.[14]

Ely's readers may have helped him briefly, but by 1813—the year Benjamin Rush died—Ely quit the New York poorhouse, exhausted and disillusioned, and took a more traditional (and paying) position as a parish minister in Philadelphia.

Some nineteenth-century sermons blame and berate the poor more starkly than others. In a sermon preached at Halifax, Nova Scotia, on Christmas Day, 1818, for example, Methodist preacher James Priestley argued, "It is the duty of the poor to be perfectly contented, and never to murmur at the dispensations of Providence."[15] The sermon was purportedly "published by request for the benefit of the poor." The poor were, Priestley insisted, "particularly obliged to be industrious lest distress should tempt them to dishonesty."[16] The rich, however, were not exempt from Priestley's sharp judgments: While they ought to live as simply as the poor, he said, the rich also have as their specific duty "to have pity on the poor."[17] This classic view that rich and poor have specific responsibilities, the one to help, the other to be dependent and industrious or grateful, is reminiscent of texts such as the *Shepherd of Hermas,* usually dated to the second century CE. This text is best known for its parable of the interdependence between the strong and powerful elm tree and the fragile but fruitful vine that survives by living on the tree's more robust structure. The parable served as a reminder of the value for mutual interdependence between social players of markedly different economic weight and power.[18]

Pity is hard to find in John Stanford's 1822 address to 140 young orphans in New York City. Stanford used Matthew 2:17–18 as the text for his sermon, the story of Herod's slaughter of the innocents. Stanford then built on this bloody biblical tale by describing to his young audience in vivid detail an orphanage fire that had, just two weeks earlier in Philadelphia, claimed the lives of twenty-two orphans just like themselves. Wagging his finger rhetorically from the pulpit, he emphasized the way these children had met their ruin, reminding his wards how distressed their own caretakers would be if it should happen to them. "You have now a powerful admonition, as from the ashes of these orphans, to remember your Creator," he preached, and "a most solemn warning to any of you who may indulge yourselves in sinful practices, or in the least impropriety of conduct which exposes you to the displeasure of the Almighty."[19] The fire and brimstone narrative concludes, without any apparent irony, by hoping that the children will continue to find their own institution to be "a monument of [divine] mercy and care."[20]

Not all nineteenth-century American public health sponsors and faith-based critics were so caustic. Congregational minister Samuel Hayes Elliott (1809–1869) preached and taught with exuberance until his health broke down, when he turned his energies to writing religious tracts. One of these was a hefty exposé on the New England poorhouse system, *New England's Chattels: or, Life in the Northern Poor House.*[21] The stories (all true, he said) were horrifying enough, but Elliott's tone throughout sought to defend the humanity of those who suffered, and condemned the injustices of their circumstances. Matthew Carey (1760–1839)— incidentally also the Philadelphia printer for Ely's 1813 *Almshouse Journal* as well as at least one edition of Rush's four-volume medical text—is another example of a public voice to raise awareness of charitable conditions and responses. Carey was one of the founding members of the Sunday School Society, as well as the first in America to print the Douay Bible. In 1829 he issued a free booklet with a title that tells the whole story: *Essays on the Public Charities of Philadelphia, Intended to Vindicate the Benevolent Societies of this City from the Charge of Encouraging Idleness, and to Place in Strong Relief, before an Enlightened Public, the Sufferings and Oppression under which the Greater Part of the Females Labour, who Depend on Their Industry for a Support for Themselves and Children.*[22]

Women writers in nineteenth-century America generally shared Elliott's and Carey's views and encouraged improved conditions. Unitarian educator Dorothea Lynde Dix, for example, toured prisons and institutions for the mentally insane, lobbying relentlessly for reform. She was not impressed with the Columbus State Penitentiary, which she visited in August 1844, during William Trevitt's tenure as prison physician. While Dix praised the Columbus prison for its clean refectory and adequate food for its nearly seven hundred residents, she criticized it for poor ventilation, lax discipline, and for being "totally deficient of the means of moral and mental culture," particularly in its lack of both appointed chaplains and books.[23] Whether a result of Dix's critique or not, the Columbus prison appointed a chaplain and launched a policy to provide prisoners with Bibles. James Finley, the Methodist chaplain appointed in 1846, who served the Columbus prison and its hospital inmates until just before the 1849 cholera epidemic, has left us a detailed record of his experiences in Columbus, with stories about many of the prisoners he met. Finley shared Dix's concern about the lack of books and through various appeals managed to gather what he considered a substantial library for the prisoners, which was, he says, much appreciated.[24] Finley does not name William Trevitt, who was likely in Texas with the army during much of Finley's service, but at least one prisoner in a letter Finley quotes from August 9, 1846, wrote, "We have also a good physician, who is not only a skillful, but a kind and Christian man."[25]

Other women writers from this era were similarly concerned with the conditions of those who lived at the social margins. Mary Jane Holmes (1825–1907), an active Episcopalian and niece of Connecticut Congregationalist preacher Joel Hawes, published thirty-nine popular novels that focus on moral justice, class, race, and gender relationships. Her book sales during her lifetime were exceeded, it was said, only by those of Harriet Beecher Stowe.[26] Many of Holmes's novels focus on the power of women's literacy and are frank in describing health risks, infant mortality, and life for the poor in the rural New England villages of the day.[27]

THE DOCTOR, THE PRESBYTERIAN MISSIONARY, AND THE AMERICAN HOSPITAL IN CHILE

Writing her family's history in the late 1800s, Sarah Jane Trevitt summarized her brother Henry's life in three concise sentences. She notes Henry's service as his uncle's clerk at the State House, then says, "In 1858 he went with his uncle to Valparaiso and had charge of the American Hospital one year. In 1860 he returned to New Hampshire and started in the practice of medicine in Wilton." How was it, I wondered, that Henry, who seemed to be the least adventurous man in his family, chose to leave Ohio and travel at considerable personal risk all the way to South America? And what made Henry qualified to direct a hospital in a foreign country? Pursuing these questions, my research into the primary public records, government documents, and other sources eventually led me to the rare books library at Princeton Seminary to consult the journals of the Reverend Dr. David Trumbull, an American Congregationalist and hospital chaplain in Chile.

Henry's and his uncle's work in Valparaiso, Chile, was part of a long history of American government service providing support, including institutionalized medical care, to suffering citizens who found themselves living as expatriates abroad, a tradition that continues in American embassies around the world today. For Trumbull and the Trevitts, those they served were for the most part hospitalized travelers and indigent sailors. Such government-funded hospitals that were associated with a country's consulate in a foreign land also often included chaplains like Trumbull, who were not government employees but served the sick poor as Christian missionaries, driven by a sense of moral urgency to preach the gospel and reach out to the local community. The American Hospital that Sarah Jane mentions in her narrative was, I eventually learned, a curious example of one such institution with both government support and missionary presence. Its story is a tale fraught with tensions among local politics, American public policy, religion, and medicine.

Trumbull, the American Hospital's leading chaplain, began his work in Chile in 1846, the year that John, suffering a toothache, was scolding Henry for dithering over his studies. Trumbull had just graduated from Princeton Seminary. He was to remain in South America, where he ministered especially to sick American sailors and émigrés, until his death in 1889. And though the mission society that sponsored him would turn over its work in Chile to the U.S. Presbyterian Church in 1872, during the Trevitts' association with him between 1858 and 1860, Trumbull was, like them—and would remain—a Congregationalist.

In the mid-nineteenth century, Chile was a strictly Roman Catholic country. Its state and church authorities frowned on Protestant missionaries and made it nearly impossible for them to influence local religious practices. In Valparaiso, for example, writes one of Trumbull's biographers:

> Public worship was forbidden. A Protestant in South America was as much lost as a man without a country. He had no church, no social position, no legal rights. Civil marriage was not allowed, and it was almost impossible for him to find a way to be married, except on board an English or American ship outside the three-mile area of sea over which a country has control. All the cemeteries were owned by the Catholic Church, and the only burial place for a Protestant in Valparaiso was the dumping ground outside the city.[28]

Against such pressures, Trumbull battled the authorities in a persistent and ultimately successful effort to establish the first Protestant church in South America, agreeing to the government's insistence that the building (which could not look like a church) be surrounded by a high fence with a small inconspicuous gate to the street, "and that hymns and anthems be sung so softly that passersby could never hear them and be tempted to step in to listen."[29] Determined to have a more public presence, Trumbull began to seek out and visit sick English-speaking sailors, who he found on the many ships that came into harbor during those years when Valparaiso was a major port on the sea route to the gold mines of California. Others who needed him he found in the city hospitals and prisons, where they often landed after a drunken spree. In response to the desperate needs he perceived, Trumbull soon opened a mission headquarters on the waterfront, marked by a flag to invite sailors inside. He also began the first Protestant newspaper in Spanish, and wrote sermons and editorials for the local Spanish papers.[30] He eventually gained such respect among Catholic authorities in Valparaiso that during a cholera epidemic he "was appointed a member of the relief committee and joined forces with the Catholics in relieving the distress of the poor and providing extra hospital space."[31]

Trumbull's pressure on the authorities to increase religious visibility for Protestant expats in Chile helped other churches in the city. St. Paul's Anglican Church, for example, which had met in a private home since 1837, launched its building program in 1858, the year the Trevitts arrived, though its builders were still forbidden to shape the edifice to *look* like a church.[32] Throughout his forty years in Chile, Trumbull kept close ties with his New England colleagues and supporters, sending his children home to college at Harvard, Yale, Wellesley, and Smith. Of his nine children, one son—John, born in 1856—would devote his career to medical service in Valparaiso.

The city's importance had skyrocketed thanks to the 1849 gold rush. While some travelers risked the brutal jungle journey by donkey trail (and by the late 1850s, trains) across the Panama isthmus, the most common route to California from the East Coast of North America was to sail south around Cape Horn in what could be a harrowing three or four month odyssey.[33] In July 1857, as Trumbull and his wife were beginning their second decade of work in Valparaiso, the newly elected US President James Buchanan appointed Dr. William Trevitt to serve as American ambassador to Chile.

The vituperative party politics of this appointment are evident in the tone of the Columbus reporter who announced the news, hinting at bitter local political tensions that perhaps led to William's lobbying for this new position. These tensions followed in part from a recent state treasury extortion scandal in Columbus, in which the state treasurer, John G. Breslin, was accused of diverting and misappropriating half a million dollars in tax funds to his own use. Public opinion blamed William (whose office was next door to Breslin's) for remaining silent when he must have known what was going on. "Dr. Trevitt has got an office," the paper announced on July 22, 1857. "Old Buck [President Buchanan] has recognized his eminent services and appointed him to be Consul at Valparaiso. This is another triumph of the Post Office clique, which seems resolved to wipe out the influence of the 'Old Wheel-horse' as fast as possible."[34] "Old Wheel-horse" referred to Samuel Medary, a Columbus newspaper publisher of the Democrat Party, who was, like Trevitt (another ardent Democrat), granted a new presidential appointment that conveniently removed him from the city and its local politics. Whether William had known about the treasury fraud or not, young Henry—who served as William's clerk during the period in question—would later face a similar public shaming for remaining silent, in his case pertaining to a suspected murder.

William was, to all appearances, delighted with the new appointment. The family, including his wife and four sons—but not at first Henry—left Columbus and sailed out of New York City on October 16, 1857, rounding Cape Horn and arriving in Valparaiso soon after the new year, on January 14, 1858.[35]

William Trevitt was, it appears from all the public records and reflections by those who knew him, a highly opinionated cyclone of a man, accustomed to quick decisions and to getting whatever he wanted, both as a doctor and a politician. He also appears to have been an excellent and much appreciated physician. He was on multiple committees of the Ohio State Medical Society and a voice in the development of ethical guidelines for qualifying physicians.[36] He was also considered (or at least considered himself) an expert on cholera.[37] In addition to his 1849 "Report on Cholera," summarizing the disease course and outcome in the prison, William published a "Letter on Cholera" that described his experience with its treatment during the 1832–1833 epidemic as well as the more recent outbreak. William's narratives about this disease that even he did not quite understand were published only a few years before Dr. John Snow's famous removal of the Broad Street pump handle in London, on Friday, September 8, 1854, an act regarded in the history of public health as the defining moment proving cholera's relationship with water-borne contamination by human waste. Trevitt's "Letter" was largely an appeal to "do no harm." He advised his medical peers to avoid harsh dosing of cholera victims in favor of prompt but moderate medical intervention. It was important, he said, that "the patient does not run the risk of being drugged to death," since "Most persons would rather die of Disease than of the Doctor."[38] Over the next decade William would also publish a treatise on medicinal spring waters,[39] promote the vaccination of penitentiary residents for smallpox,[40] and use his long sea voyage to Chile as an opportunity to write about travel medicine and effective treatments for seasickness, in three letters that his friends and colleagues back at Starling quickly published for the medical community.[41]

William was also known for his quick-temper. Dr. Wilhelm Trevitt Knappe (b. 1845), a physician who later considered William one of his teachers and whose father had worked with him in political office, would claim that William once traveled to Springfield Illinois intent on challenging Abraham Lincoln to a duel—most likely during Lincoln's tenure in the House of

Representatives starting in 1846—for "trying in every way to starve our soldiers in Mexico."[42]

A force of nature in Ohio, William Trevitt as America's ambassador to Chile quickly got himself into trouble in Valparaiso, alienating resident expatriates, both his fellow Americans and their neighbors. The crisis culminated in a spectacular standoff with a contingent of soldiers from the Chilean government during a revolution in February and March 1859 that led to expulsion from his post and a scandal that was to reverberate in the newspapers and the congressional record in Washington, DC, for decades.

It began soon after William arrived in Chile as the new Consul. The American Hospital was a facility officially under the jurisdiction of the US government, which paid, on a contract system, a fixed rate per day per patient for its care of Americans far from home who found themselves sick and in need of medical attention. While most patients were sick sailors, the hospital was also available to all travelers who had nowhere else to stay during an illness. There were similar facilities in the city at this time for English and German travelers and seamen, and the city also had a number of public and private Chilean hospitals.[43]

For many years the US government's Valparaiso contract for the American Hospital had been held by Dr. Thomas Page, who operated the hospital in a facility he had established on his personal property. For reasons that remain unclear, soon after his arrival in the city, William Trevitt chose to revoke Page's contract, and to relocate the American Hospital to facilities under his own control. He summoned Henry, still in Columbus, to join him in Chile and take over its direction. It must have seemed a golden career opportunity for Henry, who hurriedly applied for a passport in May of 1858 but could not arrive in the city earlier than the fall of that year.[44] Some weeks after his arrival, a fire destroyed much of downtown Valparaiso on November 13, 1858, including the Trevitts' residence and all of their personal property. The disaster so affected one of William's sons that the boy spiraled into a mental breakdown that would plague him and his family for years to come. A *New York Times* correspondent summarized these family affairs for stateside friends in January 1859:

> A son of the American Consul, Dr. Trevitt, has been suffering from an attack of insanity for some weeks. . . . The American Hospital has recently passed out of the hands of Dr. Page, who has had it for many years, nearly twenty, into the care of a nephew of the Consul, also called Dr. Trevitt, who arrived a few months ago from Ohio. Dr. T. No. 1, the Consul, was . . . among the recent sufferers by the fire.[45]

William's dismissal of the respected Dr. Thomas Page in favor of an unknown young nephew outraged the local expatriate community, although the newspaper accounts of this reaction consistently cite William rather than blaming Henry for the resulting difficulties and conditions. William's motives for forcing such a public insult are unclear. It is possible that he had known Page during their medical school years in Philadelphia in the early 1830s. And in fact Page's medical care had not impressed every traveler to Valparaiso. In 1850 a Miss Ellen M. Knights, writing home to Boston about her safe arrival in Valparaiso, said of Page's hospital that "Bitter complaints are made of the American Hospital here. It certainly is a most miserable place. The sailors say [i]t is shure [*sic*] death to a man to go there."[46]

William initially moved the site of the American Hospital from its base on Page's personal property to his own residence, a large villa, known as the "house of the Venegas," located a short distance outside of town high in the hills.[47] But on the night of February 28, 1859, a political uprising that had been brewing across the country broke out in a revolutionary attack on the palace of the governor (the intendente) in Valparaiso. Armed citizens attacked the palace and, blocked by guards from forcible entry, used gunfire and attempted to set the place on fire. They then seized arms stored in the Custom House; what followed was a bloody gunfight in the municipal square. William's downtown consular office was nearby and his secretary, Charles Rand, would later note that the government's gunfire on the day of the revolution had damaged the building, the flag, and passed "within an inch of a lady who had fled to the office for protection." Describing what followed, one reporter wrote:

> [T]he ammunition of the insurgents giving out after an hour's fight, they retreated among the ravines and dispersed . . . From what I have seen I think that from 100 to 150 must have been killed and wounded. One of the leaders, named Villar, was shot this morning; another named Fierre, has been sentenced to death but allowed to appeal; a third, Riobo, has taken refuge in the house of the American Consul, but will have to be given up . . . All the foreign houses are closed, business of course at a standstill.[48]

The Chilean government's response was immediate and forceful. Police and soldiers began to make the rounds of all private homes, respecting no one's privacy and (it was reported) pillaging indiscriminately and killing a number of American and British residents in cold blood. Two days later, on March 2, they arrived at the American consulate.

Our best source for what happened next is a first-person narrative that Rand, a native of Philadelphia who was also fluent in Spanish, wrote immediately following the events themselves.[49] Rand was present with the Trevitts throughout the revolution and the invasion of the consulate that followed, and his account, later published in a number of American papers, describes incidents as they happened (apart from a brief period when he was knocked unconscious).

According to Rand, "thirty or forty" frightened local citizens sought refuge in the American Hospital on February 28, many of them safely departing to their homes within a day or two. Those who stayed included six men, including Bartolome and Damian Riobo, who were later seized and taken into custody as suspected instigators in the February revolution. According to one report, "Rand was a particular friend and associate of one of the Riobos, who was a reporter for the *Mercurio* [Valparaiso's most powerful newspaper], and it was Rand whose advice led the Consul into the scrape."

The scrape itself took place on the afternoon of March 2. A contingent of government soldiers, acting on reports that Riobo (most likely Bartolome, later condemned to death) had been seen strolling along an upstairs porch of the Trevitt's consular villa, scaled a wall and took control of the front gate, then entered the building to demand that the dissidents be handed over for arrest and trial. When the soldiers first arrived, Rand says, he and William, with "Dr. Henry Trevitt, his nephew," were on the road a short distance away, approaching the house from the consulate's office in the city. In William's absence his wife Lucinda, faced with "eighteen or twenty" armed men and their chief officer at the door, had attempted a delay by doing the only thing she could think of "for protection against insult": she took an American flag and flung it down across the entry steps, dramatically daring the soldiers to violate the sanctuary of its symbolic fabric at their own risk. Unfortunately this theatrical patriotic act, which was to make headlines across America, failed. The captain took the dare, marched across the flag, and seized control of the building. Once inside, Rand reports, the captain

> sat down and wrote a note to the Governor of Valparaiso, stating that *by mistake* he found himself in the premises of the American Consul, and that he had seen there a gentleman suspected of being compromised in the tumult of the 28th February, asking whether he should arrest him, that Mrs. Trevitt would not permit him to do so.

Clearly Rand did not believe the visit was a mistake, although this was also how Trumbull would hear the news. Such an error was impossible, Rand insisted, because "[d]uring the affair of the 2d the American flag was displayed upon a flagstaff from the dwelling where it had been flying ever since the day of the revolution (28th of Feb.)." Rand and the Trevitts reached the gate shortly after this note was dispatched to the governor.

William was incensed at being initially barred from entering his own gate. Once inside, he became livid when his wife, Rand says, "came upon the balcony over head and called to Dr. Trevitt, telling him that there was an armed man in her room who called himself an officer and who had been very insolent to her." Rushing upstairs, William threw himself into battle, attempting to disarm the captain of his sword while Rand and Mrs. Trevitt tried to bar the soldiers' access to the stairway. While William's fifteen-year-old son, Willie, helped to block the doors, Henry disappears from the story entirely. After the captain was disarmed, a message arrived from the governor that supported him, asking "if there was any impediment to their delivery to be tried." William sued for time, persuading the armed contingent to leave, and wrote to the governor the next morning "stating the outrage committed upon his residence" and insisting that before he could do anything he must first consult with the American government's "Minister Plenipotentiary."

The next day, Rand says, "a large body of military . . . halted in front of the house . . . with a note from the Governor, demanding the surrender of the supposed offenders, mentioning one of them by name." In the presence of a visiting notary public there on purpose to record William's official objections, and several other American officials, the Chilean commander told William that the soldiers' orders were to take the local rebels who had sought asylum in the consulate "at whatever cost; that he had brought a force sufficiently large to do it; and that he would be compelled to do it, even if he had to *fire the house*." Anxious to avoid "the effusion of blood," William conceded defeat, allowed a house search for the suspects, and "declared his intention of committing his protest to paper and abandoning his dwelling to the military."

Rand's letter ends with a heart-rending appeal for those who had been arrested. "They came," he says,

> flying from the reckless cruelties committed by the victorious troops on the 28th of February, as did thirty or forty others—the residence of the Consul being upon the hills some ¾ of a mile from the city proper. . . . Humanity forbade their being turned out to meet with almost certain death—there was no evidence nor even accusation presented against any or either of them, verbal or written, official or otherwise, until *after* the outrage of the 2nd ins., and that outrage was and *is yet* unatoned for.

The crisis cost William his appointment. On March 4, 1859, the government of Chile revoked Trevitt's "exequatur" or legal privilege to serve as consul in Chile, putting him out of a job. The Trevitts were allowed to leave the building safely, and the American government quickly authorized the vice consul to serve in William's place. Although there is some evidence that William made at least one quick trip back to the United States that summer,[50] in fact the Trevitts would continue to make Valparaiso their home base for another year, until February 1860, when William got a new appointment, as consul to Peru.

During this interim year, the American Hospital in Valparaiso, which the Trevitts still directed, was located in a rented building downtown near the wharf. It continued to be criticized for substandard care,[51] even though the fiscal records suggest it was amply funded from Washington. Throughout 1859 and early 1860, William continued to bill the US government for all expenses related to medical care, and he also claimed a portion of his salary as US consul. Officials in Washington were to take more than a decade to sort out these financial claims, including an audit of his apparently chaotic expense reports.[52] William would eventually recoup more than eight thousand dollars that he said he spent on aid for sick Americans who received their care at the Hospital; he lost the bid for his salary. Although Henry was officially in charge of the hospital during this year (the records are vague on what portion of William's claim might have paid Henry's salary), Henry is treated in the official documents as an unnamed underling, with no association (on paper at least) with his uncle's financial tangles.

Throughout this political debacle, David Trumbull, for one, was less than impressed with the new Consul. Trumbull's private journal cites at least one awkward encounter, in December 1858, when Trumbull learned after the fact that William had expected him to preside at a funeral that morning; he jotted this down and noted that he sent William an apology. On March 8, 1859, referring to the attack on the consulate a few days earlier, Trumbull wrote, "read new consp[iracy] with U.S. Consul ab't soldiers going to his house—said sent officer to English Hospital, who made mistake and went to American."[53]

The Trumbulls' diaries are as friendly toward the ousted Dr. Page as they are brief and clipped in reference to William. Page had many local friends and supporters, including Trumbull's wife, Jane, who had depended on Page as her physician during the delivery of most of their children.[54] The Trumbulls also heartily welcomed the doctor who eventually took over the hospital after the Trevitts left Chile in 1860, Dr. James Aquinas Ried, a native of Bavaria who had been in Valparaiso since 1844.[55] Page for his part refused to accept his abrupt loss of the government's lucrative contract to provide medical care for American sailors. In 1861, well rid of the Trevitts, Page submitted a new bid to the US government to run the Hospital once again,[56] and by 1863 he had it back. In a March letter from Valparaiso, Trumbull reports to his mission, with palpable relief, that "Dr. Page has the destitute American Seamen again in his hospital. They are comfortable now; the quarters are good." Affirming Trumbull's satisfaction in June a year later, James Muller, a Bible evangelist for Trumbull's Presbyterian mission to sailors, reported that Trumbull once again "holds religious services once or twice a week in one of the wards of the American Hospital, and speaks of the great kindness of Dr. Page, the Surgeon of this Hospital."[57]

Thomas Page was not young and his victory was brief; in 1869 he moved permanently to California, where he died in 1872.[58] The American Hospital in Valparaiso closed its doors permanently with his departure. An 1871 report by a subsequent consul at Valparaiso, J. C. Caldwell, noted that

> At this city there was formerly an American Hospital, but this has now been abandoned . . . [I]n my opinion, judging from the extraordinary expenditures on account of medical aid, the place was either used improperly or else was not in the least economically administered. Any of the accounts given in this communication before 1870 will show the absurdity of the expenses . . . plainly indicat[ing] to my mind that under former consuls, in many instances, there was gross negligence or irregularity in the disposition of the fund for the relief of destitute American sailors at this port . . . The present Consul uses the English hospital.[59]

The Page family would continue to play a prominent role in the Valparaiso medical community. Thomas Page's son Olof, who, like his father and William Trevitt, studied medicine in Philadelphia, would become, fifty years later, "one of the most prominent practitioners of the city" and the leading surgeon in Valparaiso's largest medical facility, the Hospital San Juan de Dios (where his monthly salary was 40 pesos, or $US10). Nicholas Senn, a Chicago physician touring South American hospitals at the turn of the twentieth century, met Olof and praised his philanthropic dedication:

> The care of the sick is in the hands of 26 Sisters of Charity, female helpers and orderlies, all of whom know little about nursing and much less about the preparation for surgical operations . . . [and] not much can be said of the neatness and

cleanliness of the institution. There would be little inducement to serve in the capacity of surgeon in such a hospital if it were not for the consciousness of doing something for the sake of charity.[60]

HENRY AT HOME: FROM PHINEAS GAGE TO THE POORHOUSE

The upheaval in Chile must have made life rather difficult for Henry Trevitt, now in his late thirties. By the time of his one-year assignment in Chile, he had been immersed in at least the social circles of American medicine and health policy for nearly twenty years, but even so he was hardly skilled in the care of wounded and drunken sailors, travelers who had been sick for months at sea without a doctor, and penniless gold diggers from California who arrived in port riddled with worms and scurvy.

For despite John's scolding, Henry had continued to put off the medical studies that his family clearly expected of him. He likely knew well many of the stories about his uncle's success as a surgeon in Texas during the Mexican-American conflict in 1846. Henry may also have been among the number of "medical students and citizens . . . engaged as attendants and nurses" who helped care for the prison's cholera victims in 1849, when "the [prison] hospital was overcrowded with the sick, the dying, and the ghastly corpses of the newly dead."[61] He was surely conversant with his uncle's research and publications on local medicinal springs, as well as his strong views on standards for medical education. He also certainly knew a great deal about bookkeeping as it related to government spending and political wrangling, and at home he was intimately familiar with William's complex property taxes and debts.[62] Henry is also named in the public records in 1857 as a notary for the state in a lawsuit between one of his uncle's medical partners, Dr. John Dawson, and a blind Columbus prisoner who charged Dawson with attacking his good eye with a surgical knife (Dawson won the case).[63] While Henry must have taken classes at Starling in order to qualify for his medical degree when he returned from South America,[64] there is in fact no evidence that he ever had a single encounter in clinical medicine as a doctor caring for the sick before he arrived in Chile.

Frankly, he viewed himself as more of an artist. Perhaps influenced by his sister's work as a landscape painter and art teacher, Henry had taken up the newest trend, daguerreotype photography. In the spring of 1848 he spent three weeks as an itinerant photographer in Fort Wayne, Indiana (perhaps curious to see a place he had heard about as a child from stories in his uncle John's letters).[65] By 1850 Henry was advertising his daguerreotype studio in the Columbus city directory. The 1850 census—which lists occupations based on what household members actually told the census workers—identifies Henry as an "Artist" living at his uncle's address.[66] Although he would return to New Hampshire with a medical microscope that had been state of the art in the early 1850s (shown, with his wife's rosary, in the photo that opens this chapter), Henry's fascination was likely in what he could see of the world through its eyepiece, rather than the opportunity it gave him to be a more effective doctor.

Henry's apparently reluctant career in early American public health medicine was also shaped by two private family tragedies. Shortly before he left for Chile, he became engaged to a woman known only from oral tradition and the gold watch case she gave him as an engagement gift, which is inscribed "to H.T. from M.A.G." Although she would die of tuberculosis before the wedding, Henry preserved among his personal effects for the rest of his life the watch with its case as well as the rings he bought her and a small oval locket of the same pattern, perhaps also hers, containing a perfectly sized oval glass ambrotype of an unknown dark-eyed woman decked in gold jewelry. We don't know when she died, but it was sometime after the summer of 1857 and before he returned home, alone, to New Hampshire late in 1860.[67]

The second tragedy was the family crisis in Valparaiso, marked by the abrupt mental illness of his young cousin, a break first triggered by the city fire of November 1858.[68] By January or February of 1859, William wrote home that family members who had "suffered considerably from illness, are nearly restored to their accustomed health." But Rand's first-person account of the Chilean government's attack on the American consulate in March claims that in fact the boy's emotionally fragile state was a key factor in William's agreement to surrender the sanctuary rebels when the soldiers threatened to set the building on fire. William gave up the prisoners (who he would have known faced a likely death sentence) because he was concerned that his son's condition, said Rand, "was likely to be seriously prejudiced by his remaining a spectator of possible scenes of violence."[69] Yet it was Henry, not William, who accompanied the boy, two of his brothers, and their mother back to the United States in early 1860, leaving William in Peru with their teenage son Willie for the following year. The fact that Henry disappears from Rand's account of the armed conflict may suggest that Henry was attending, as a resident physician, to the care of this disturbed son.

Back in Ohio, Henry stayed in Columbus only briefly, to settle his aunt and cousins at home, to catch up with friends and colleagues at Starling, and to (finally) receive his medical degree. During these short weeks, perhaps in October or early November of 1860, Henry attended a medical meeting where he made a short public comment that was to attest his presence, at least, in the annals of American medicine. The comment concerned a man named Phineas Gage (see Figure 3.3).

Gage, who had been a railroad worker in Vermont, was well known by 1860 as a medical legend. In 1848 he had nearly died in a railway accident when an explosion blasted a thirteen-pound, four-foot-long iron tamping rod through his skull.[70] He lost an eye, but to everyone's surprise, recovered. The doctors were especially interested in learning from this "natural experiment" how the accident affected his brain, and this neurologic fascination with Gage has continued to the present.[71] By 1859 the recovered

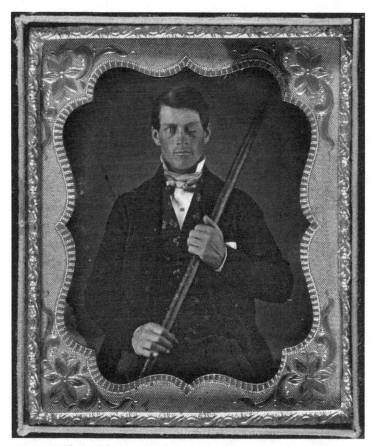

FIGURE 3.3 Phineas Gage in the 1850s, seen here with the inscribed iron tamping rod that pierced his head and removed his eye in a Vermont railroad accident in 1848. The image has been laterally reversed to show the features correctly since daguerreotypes are mirror images. From the collection of Jack and Beverly Wilgus. Used with permission.

Gage had left New England, gone into the circus where for a time he made a public spectacle of his injury and the iron rod, then sailed south to work with horses as a stagecoach driver on the roads between Chile and Peru. It was there that he met Henry Trevitt. When Gage's name came up during a medical meeting at Starling in the fall of 1860, and someone wondered aloud what had happened to him, those keeping notes at the meeting would later report that

> Dr. Henry Trevitt, of Valparaiso, South America, who was present, at once replied to our remark that he knew Gage well; that he lived in Chili [*sic*], where he was engaged in stage driving; and that he was in the enjoyment of good health, with no impairment whatever of his mental faculties.[72]

This published record is all that we know about Henry's interactions with Gage in South America. But the encounter between the two men somewhere on the high plateau of roads in a foreign country—where stagecoach was the common transport—was surely yet another chapter in Henry's medical education on the social consequences of aberrant cases and illnesses. Indeed these experiences—from epidemic and chronic disease to the mental afflictions of prisoners, stagecoach drivers, and young affluent doctors' sons alike—were to clearly shape his subsequent career and personal encounters on his return to the United States, although we cannot know how they shaped his personal thinking.

Nor do we know why Henry returned home to New Hampshire in 1860 after twenty years in Ohio. It may be that the political and family crisis, together with his involvement in hospital administration and conditions that all sources suggest were abysmal under William Trevitt, had caused some break with his uncle. There is no evidence that they ever met again. Perhaps Henry simply wanted to make a new beginning after his fiancée died. Or perhaps his return marked a family decision related to his father's death late in the summer of 1858, likely while Henry was traveling to South America. There is also no evidence that the Civil War played any role in Henry's activities in 1860 or later. Indeed the only sign of the Civil War era among his surviving effects is a small U.S. Army medicine pannier, an iron-bound wooden doctor's trunk of a type that did not become popular until 1860, and was used by army physicians throughout the Civil War. The trunk likely belonged to John, who in the early days of the Civil War was briefly captured at New Orleans in the spring of 1860, on his way home to Mont Vernon from his final Army post in Texas. By 1861 John had retired and, newly married, was living together with their mother and Sarah Jane, growing strawberries and serving as legal executor to help settle a number of local citizens' estates. It was John who would continue a relationship with William and his family, in fact coming to William's rescue to buy his uncle's Columbus home when William, aging and ill, declared bankruptcy in 1877.[73]

At some point in 1861, Henry moved to the village of Wilton, renting a room in the local hotel while establishing himself in the practice of medicine. There were of course already several other doctors in town; to make a living and perhaps because he thought it would be fun, Henry opened a drugstore that would eventually include one of the town's first ice cream soda machines. He was to live in Wilton for the next thirty years, doing business as the town druggist, practicing as an occasional consulting physician for his neighbors, and caring for the health of those marginalized by homelessness, mental illness, and social poverties. By the late 1860s, he was appointed physician to the residents of the local poorhouse, thus becoming an "overseer of the poor," one of the officials who directed the nineteenth-century public welfare system in America. It was likely here in southern New Hampshire sometime during the years that followed, when Seth Saltmarsh's copy of Benjamin Rush's text found its way into his permanent library. It would be the only book in his library that Henry's wife Ellen, many years later, would pack into the small wicker trunk of family memories that eventually made its way into my grandmother's room.

Henry's experiences as a public medical and government clerk in Ohio and as a doctor in Chile had prepared him sufficiently to care for the local sick poor in New England. At least the

local welfare officials thought so. An 1869 county commissioners'
report made it a point to name him and "speak in complimentary
terms" of his services. The commissioners also leave us a list of
Henry's roughly one hundred patients at the Wilton poorhouse.
They included "29 harmless insane, 7 requiring close confine-
ment, and 10 idiots," according to the report, which notes further that "Most of the remaining 64 are feeble, with impaired or
broken constitutions, unable to perform much productive labor;
demanding dilligence [sic] and constant care to attend to their
legitimate wants."[74] The poorhouse—a new building that consoli-
dated a population that had previously been scattered across the
county—also doubled as a low-security prison. The 1870 census
lists their diagnoses using such labels as "idiotic," "insane," "ine-
briate," "blind," "simple," and "sentenced for drunkenness."

Attending physicians who served the county poorhouse were
responsible for providing at best very basic medical services: they
visited the sick, attended and attested births, advised on medications, and issued death certificates. Medical fees for these services
were paid from public tax income.

A report from Dr. Samuel Gridley Howe of the Board of
Charities in Massachusetts in 1867, contemporary with Henry's
work in neighboring New Hampshire, emphasizes the prevailing
moral ethics of such public service. Howe's comments also indicate how many still regarded the American Revolution as a recent
event that shaped community ideals:

> The purpose of charity in New England has been to diminish
> the number of the helpless, to make them sounder, stronger,
> more hopeful and self-reliant. Justice, no less than mercy, has
> been in the thoughts of our people: a justice not satisfied with
> almsgiving, but seeking zealously to establish a social condi-
> tion in which alms would be less and less needed. Painful as the
> sights of woe in many of our charitable institutions might be,
> they are made more tolerable by the thought that in America—
> the home of the poor man—we are in the way to throw off and

neutralize much of the misery handed down to us from older countries and less hopeful times.[75]

Despite Howe's optimism, it is not clear that misery was in fact quite so readily thrown off at the Wilton poorhouse. According to the 1869 Wilton Commissioners' Report, half of the twenty-six residents who had died during 1868 were victims of tuberculosis, too weak to resist the misery of disease and poverty, and requiring public alms to the end of their lives. Indeed tuberculosis—another epidemic of Henry's era that faces us now again with the drug-resistant forms of the twenty-first century—would claim the lives of all three of Henry and Ellen's daughters in quick succession only a few years later. Ellen alone would hang on into her 90s, outliving them all until 1945, her last days spent in the house of a stranger as a ward of the state under Roosevelt's new system of social security and public welfare.

MURDER, MATERNAL MORTALITY, AND SMALL-TOWN GOSSIP

But all that was far in the future when Henry moved to Wilton in 1861. The first challenge he faced in the village was not disease but murder. His work included delivering babies and writing death certificates for ordinary town citizens, not just poorhouse residents. Obstetrics often overlapped with forensics in a relationship that was not always what it seemed. When twelve-year-old Ida Major—legally married, if only for a few weeks—gave birth to her first child in late 1869, it was Henry who attended the birth at her parents' home; the infant quickly died. Much later, Henry would remember that earlier that year, in March, Elwin Major— who seduced Ida while working as a farm laborer for her father— had come into Henry's pharmacy to buy strychnine, telling the druggist he wanted it to kill foxes. Henry was vaguely troubled that fall when Ida's older sister Ella, an unmarried schoolteacher also rumored to be pregnant, died in strange circumstances.

Two years later, when Ida's third child died quickly with no apparent cause, Henry's suspicions deepened, but still he kept them to himself.[76] He could not prove foul play, and his years as a notary and clerk in Ohio for physicians at the prison and the State House had schooled him well in legal silence. It was not until Ida herself died in 1874, at age eighteen, in inexplicable agony during labor with her fifth child, that Henry—now newly married to Ellen, a vibrant young accountant half his age—chose to speak out. "I thought it time to make the facts known when an investigation was made," he later told the court at Major's trial for murder by strychnine poisoning. Many in the village blamed Ida's death (and Ella's) on Henry's silence, even though Major stubbornly insisted that Ida had poisoned herself with a camphor overdose. The dead girl's nearest neighbor insisted that the Majors had been a happy couple, since, she remembered, Ida "always did as he said, and chopped wood and carried water."[77] The first jury could not agree, but at the second trial the medical evidence was clear enough, and Major was hanged for his crime, at Concord in 1877. Henry was a witness for the prosecution. In his final decision, the judge made it a point to emphasize that while some might think Henry a scoundrel for his long silence, in the view of the court Henry was not at fault for Ida's death. Still, surviving Wilton town records suggest a marked drop in Henry's public welfare income in the years following the trial. Henry weathered his unpopularity with stoic cheer, buying exotic fruit (like bananas) for his shop and stocking up on popular patent medicines. His oldest daughter Carita, forced to spend a year behind the shop counter after high school before she went back to school as a teacher, found the store immensely dull, devoting her time to darning her father's socks and writing letters. Ellen, seared by town gossip over the trial, took the train—and often the children—to visit her family in Boston as often as she could. The children grew up never to speak any ill of their father, delighting instead in art lessons, photography, and the first ice cream sodas of every summer. As Henry turned seventy, he began to wander the village absentmindedly, but he could still set a child's broken bones, lending his daughters books, and rejoicing whenever they arrived home from their frequent travels. And on a shelf somewhere in the gabled and turreted house Henry had built at the top of Bales Hill Road, Seth Saltmarsh's copy of Benjamin Rush's medical text sat waiting, ready for its next consultation.

CIVIC DUTY, RELIGION, AND THE GIFT

I chose to tell Henry's story in this chapter as an example of and glimpse into nineteenth-century medical interactions with civic life, religion, and politics as they shaped the way that many Americans thought and spoke of care for the poor. Admittedly, religion plays an almost silent role in Henry's own story, although we do know that both he and his uncle William faithfully attended church throughout their lives. In Peru, for example, William actively supported the same Presbyterian "seamen's mission" that Trumbull served in Chile.[78] In New Hampshire, Henry's relatives were all Congregationalists; he and Ellen were married by Wilton's Congregational-Unitarian minister. While Henry frequently accompanied their children to a variety of different town worship services and religious events, there is no hint that his wife ever attended church. Indeed, Ellen was baptized only when she converted to Roman Catholicism in her eighties, a move that shocked her descendants' staunch Congregationalist families to their socks.[79] Her father was a nominal Protestant and few acquaintances would have guessed that all of her maternal Canadian relatives were lifelong devout Catholics; it was one of these distant nieces who was instrumental in her late conversion. Protestant-Catholic "mixed" marriages were often kept secret in this era, and her parents' move to Boston before or early in their marriage doubtless helped keep things quiet. As for Henry's family, it seems, religion was at most a civic responsibility, with Henry's public health encounters supporting a stolid sense of moral and community duty that marked the liberal religious norms of his era. American public health activities into the mid-twentieth century were built on the foundation of such lives: ordinary village doctors who found their choices shaped by and shaping particular social, political, and religious views about poverty and community health.

Henry's career is hardly an ideal model for social justice today. Indeed, his life and that of many of the other poorhouse preachers, politicians, medical teachers, and public health doctors described in this chapter give us a glimpse of what both health-care providers and those in cross-cultural faith-based aid today often work hard to avoid and prevent. They illustrate what may seem curious examples of a colonialist or patronizing approach to international relations, economic opportunism, turning a blind eye to injustices, corruption, and poor accountability, and commodification of the poor for commercial and judicial gain that at best paid lip service to religious ideals. Such tendencies in this relatively recent history of American health policy matter today because, while medical science has vastly improved, many of these social ills continue to challenge ethical, social, and economic responses not only within America but also as they relate to American health policy and tensions in humanitarian aid activities, including those of religious organizations, around the world.

This need not suggest that civic accountability—or to use the theme running through this book the "beholden-ness" of public service to the poor—is necessarily wrong or inevitably problematic. Health care for the poor in Henry's day included a commitment to a sort of civic beneficence or "gifting" (a concept explored further in Chapter 6) that remains a vital and intrinsic ingredient in virtually all societies around the world. Medical services and national ministries of health are often driven by ideals of a civic obligation to provide care free to those who most need it so long as they meet certain qualifications of entitlement (explored further in Chapter 4).

Rather, Henry's story may offer us a glimpse into the soul of much of American philanthropy today, as it views other cultures as well as the problems of poverty and health disparities within our own. Henry's experiences in what was to become the field of public health marked a hapless, almost accidental journey. His personal choices—as far as we know anything about them—seem driven not by some inner urge to serve the poor but rather by family circumstance and pressures to honor his Yankee principle to make the best show possible in life—and to prove that he could earn his own living in a profession that brought him no glory and nothing but trouble. Much that he valued, including his first love and virtually all of his personal papers, were lost in his lifetime by disaster or disease. Not only were his account books lost by the time of the Major trial, but by the end of his life all record of his personal voice was also curiously absent from the family documents and goods that his wife would box up when the Wilton house was sold in 1905. This is especially curious because Ellen herself kept meticulous records and journals—many of which have survived—but in these documents she never speaks of her husband. One suspects this April-October marriage was not a great success. "Mama thinks that the people who marry when young are always the happiest couples," their daughter Carita would write to her own fiancé in 1900, two years after Henry's death. "She thinks it is much easier for them to adjust themselves and their dispositions before they get too stubborn and set."[80] It is through such human differences, and the everyday experiences of very ordinary people, that global intersections among culture, religion, justice, and health take life.

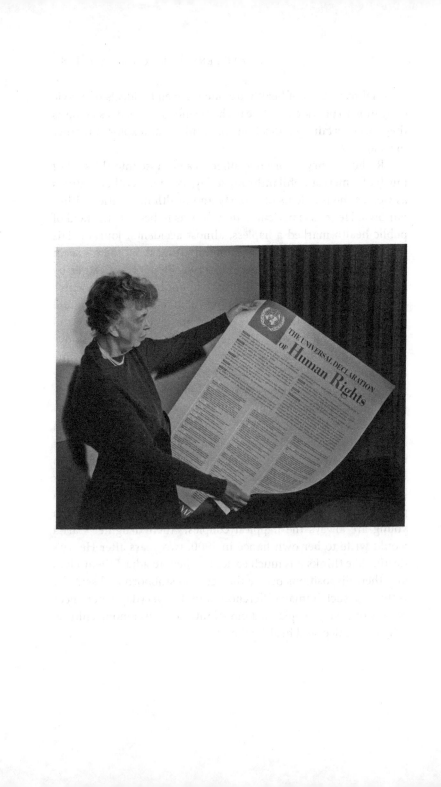

FROM MATTHEW 25

TO ARTICLE 25

Why ESC Rights Matter

ONE OF MY heroes is Daniel Barenboim, a world-class pianist and co-founder, with the late Edward Said, of the West-Eastern Divan Orchestra, one of the most acclaimed youth orchestras in the world. Each summer it draws together young talented musicians from Palestine, Israel, and other countries of the Middle East to create what Barenboim calls "musical counterpoint." The musicians who win a place in the orchestra come from many different economic, religious, and political positions, and bring with them a wide range of technical skills and formal training. Since the first summer, in 1999, some members of the orchestra have launched similar programs for children in their home countries and played in settings from Ramallah to Morocco, Germany, South America, and beyond. The orchestra is praised as "a beacon of hope on the dismal political landscape of the Middle East."[1] It seeks, says Barenboim, "to allow our curiosity and knowledge to help us inspire and create the conditions for a better future."[2] The original vision for the orchestra developed out of the friendship between Barenboim, a Jew born in Argentina and raised in Israel, and Said, an Arab Christian public intellectual and literary post-colonial theorist with roots and loyalties in Palestine. Religious differences define much of the tension that orchestra students face—in themselves and others—as they learn to play music together. Until Said's death of leukemia in 2003, his participation in the group's intentional discussions about peace despite differences was a powerful inspiration to students who were meeting—often for the very first time—people of their own age from countries they viewed as political and religious enemies.

Music is, of course, Barenboim admits, "incapable of bringing peace to the Middle East." The ruling principle is rather to shape space so that:

> a subversive accompanimental voice can enhance a melody rather than detract from it. To this day, we do not try to diminish or soften our differences in the orchestra: We do the opposite: By confronting our differences, we attempt to understand the logic behind the opposite position.[3]

Daniel Cohen, an Israeli violinist and conductor, joined the orchestra one summer in his teens. Cohen remembers the shock that he experienced during a guest session with Dr. Mustafa Barghouti, a physician and Palestinian politician and activist who is committed to nonviolence. Barghouti was explaining why the Palestinians so often experience Israeli peace and land offers as insults. Cohen recalls Barghouti telling the group, "All you Israelis talk to us as if we want something of yours, and you give it to us as if we have no right to it, you give it to us like a handout."[4] For the first time in his life, Cohen realized how even what he might think of as a generous gift was viewed, by his Muslim and Christian Palestinian neighbors, as not a gift at all but something stolen, belonging by right to those who might even still possess the property deed and house keys of homes they had been forced to abandon.

"Whether they have that right or not is not the point," said Cohen, "although I obviously think that they do." Rather, the exchange opened his eyes to the difference between charity and human rights. He saw in an instant the troubling political consequences of addressing human rights issues through a framework that those in power offered as charity. A solution, he saw, was not in whether or how much land he as a member of the dominant state might *give* to Barghouti, as a representative of the Palestinian "other." Instead, Cohen insisted, "The only thing that would be acceptable would be my coming to terms with his *right* to govern any percentage of that territory. This [realization] had a huge effect on me and my way of thinking . . . I got very upset with him and he got very upset with me, but afterwards he sat next to us at the table and we ate together."[5] Cohen's conversation with Barghouti helped him see the difference between religiously motivated charity and a position also compatible with religion that could embrace the ideas of human rights to real resource exchange in poor communities around the world and across history.

Whether we agree with Cohen or not—and regardless of what we think of contemporary politics in the Middle East—this story illustrates clearly the distinction between offers of generosity that look like charity and a human rights–based approach, the subject of this chapter. I will argue that those who work in and with religious groups may be able to engage with health workers and others concerned about social justice more effectively if they have at least a basic understanding of what the phrase "human rights" means as it relates to health and poverty. This basic understanding should include knowing what economic, social, and cultural (ESC) rights *are* in the international agreements that affect almost every country in the world today (including the United States). It should also include knowing the *history* of these agreements and why they have become so important for public policy and social justice. Furthermore, it should include knowing *how* to speak using the language of human rights with those who hold other views on religion, culture, and the ethics of entitlement.

UNDERSTANDING WHY HUMAN RIGHTS MATTER

This chapter is intended for readers who know little to nothing about the complex field of health and human rights, a field where most experts are lawyers, physicians, or advocates in health-care policy. It is vital for a number of reasons, I believe, that those who hold a religious or faith perspective and work on problems of poverty must have at least a basic understanding of human rights issues as they relate to aid for the poor. It is important first, for solidarity: because faith matters to the large majority of people who are poor in this world. It is important because a vast majority of health-care activities in poverty settings have religious roots and staff who belong to religious organizations. It is important because there is a stereotype that religion does a lot of damage, that it too often justifies the violation of human rights and human dignity. It is important because there is at least a little truth to this stereotype. It is important because, I believe, it is up to the people of faith and the people who work within such organizations to change this. Persons of faith active in poverty responses often get frustrated by the roadblocks that seem to pop up at every turn when they try to effect lasting changes to promote justice. Understanding international human rights law related to economic, social, and cultural issues relevant to health can equip newly responsive and informed choices for alternative action. Finally, an ability to understand why human rights matters is important because it can be a valuable tool in deciding what actions might be helpful or not helpful in a given situation.

Whether we think about poverty relief through a response framework of charity—based on ideas such as mercy, kindness, neighborly "love," and generous sharing—or a human rights framework that affirms social justice—based on a commitment to address and correct systematic wrongs as injustices—will depend on our view of who owns what and why. Our view will depend on our politics, our sense of self and family, and our religion. Our view will fundamentally depend on how we view the claims of human beings in need, and—if we are persons of religious faith—how we view the claims of the one we call God concerning the resources—tangible and intangible—that we find within our power.

A survey in the 1990s identified a chasm between, on the one hand, "relatively secular professionals and intellectuals oriented to universal human rights" and, on the other, "religious leaders familiar with their own traditions but less familiar with human rights in the international arena."[6] As Sumner Twiss, a religion scholar and ethicist, observed, "There is unquestionably a wide-spread perception that universal human rights are in significant tension with religious, moral, and cultural diversity in the world . . . [and yet] no persuasive case has been made to show that human rights conceived as a goal for all peoples is either illegitimate or unattainable."[7] Pulitzer Prize–winning journalist Nicholas Kristof agrees: "[R]eligious people and secular people alike do fantastic work on humanitarian issues—but they often don't work together because of mutual suspicions. If we could bridge this 'God gulf,' we would make far more progress on the world's ills."[8] No matter where we may find ourselves in this "God gulf," the conversation between Cohen and Barghouti can remind us that really working to understand the "other's" viewpoint will affirm our own human integrity and counter the risk of compromising the inner balance of all that makes us fully human.

The claim that humans have a "right" to something (such as essential food, medicine, or shelter) can be both a moral/ethical claim (based on beliefs about intrinsic human value) and a legal claim (based on specific enforceable laws). Those who focus on social justice and public health often use language about "rights" to appeal broadly to moral/ethical principles that may (or may not) align with an existing law on the books of that country or spelled out in an international covenant or treaty. And yet because a "right" sometimes can only be realized through the legislative action of a court of law, true social justice depends, ultimately, on the public sector as the "'final guarantor' of basic rights."[9] In other words, says Catholic anthropologist Dr. Paul Farmer:

> [O]nly governments can confer rights. The right to health care and the right to education can be moved forward by people like us, but non-governmental organizations, universities, foundations, and forward-thinking businesses are not, alas, in the business of conferring rights. And without basic rights—to water, security, health care, the right not to starve—then the world's poor do not have hope of a future.[10]

This split between moral/ethical and legal rights—as well as the way that economic, social, and cultural (ESC) rights are treated differently (especially in the United States) from civic and political rights (discussed further below) may at times have a direct effect on faith-based social justice activities. If we cannot press for these things in terms of national rights, and if then providing the poor with such basic essentials becomes possible only through acts shaped as charity or moral justice that lack legal power or bite, we may agree with Johannes Morsink that "It is hard to see how, for example, anyone can enjoy the right to free speech if he or she is homeless, has not eaten for days, is looking in a garbage can for a winter coat, and has not received treatment for advancing diabetes."[11]

WHAT ARE HUMAN RIGHTS?

What are human rights all about, really? How do they relate to spiritual identity, to acts in the world shaped by people of faith?

Human rights are usually connected with religion in two very different sorts of conversations. One is where we talk about the *right to religion*, that is, the right to choose or practice a religion, the right to keep religion and state separate, and so forth.[12]

The other is about a faith-based *view of human rights*. This chapter fits within this second approach, but focuses more narrowly on a group of very particular rights and how they connect to health-related problems of poverty and injustice. The discussion here further narrows in on the responses by those who work from a position (personal or organizational) that is shaped and informed by the Christian tradition. And yet, by focusing on this aspect of Western tradition that is most prevalent in aid efforts around the world today, I hope the exploration might also serve those who care about these issues from other faith-based positions.

Almost any discussion about human rights—particularly as they relate to religion and social justice—quickly becomes a minefield of debate over different views, meanings, approaches, and types of rights. The most literal meaning of a right is legislative: something guaranteed and protected by specific written law. Such laws sometimes distinguish between legal rights that protect a society's political and judicial system *from* abuses (such as military or political terrorism) and talk about rights of the poor and hungry *to* things like goods, services, and basic human dignity. Rights that protect *from* are sometimes called negative rights because they stand against something undesirable and are about *not* doing something; rights that further action and entitlement *to* something good are, in contrast, logically enough, sometimes called positive rights. Clearly, in an ordered society, it is important to have both positive and negative rights to keep away what is harmful and to ensure restorative justice. There is a common view that negative rights refer exclusively to what are called civil and political rights—for example, freedom of speech, freedom from slavery, property rights—and that positive rights are those that are called economic, social, and cultural (ESC) rights—for example, rights to food, housing, health, and employment. But this is a false dichotomy, since there need to be both negative and positive aspects to both groups of rights. ESC rights—the focus in this chapter because they concern health—are positive because enforcing them usually mandates some specific social or economic action (e.g., food, housing), but they are also negative rights in that they work to help guard against violence and injustices (e.g., food theft, forced eviction) that rob people of things that are also viewed around the world and throughout history as basic human entitlements.[13]

Another common but misleading view in legal discussions about human rights is the idea of generations of rights, with first-generation rights somehow more "legitimate" than what are called second and third-generation rights. These phrases took shape in the mid-twentieth century during the creation of the Universal Declaration of Human Rights (UDHR), discussed in more detail later.[14] Civil and political rights are sometimes called first-generation rights because, it was argued, they were the foundation laid by the eighteenth-century Enlightenment in the birth of democracy in the West, while ESC rights are called second generation because (it is claimed) they entered human rights law only later, in the nineteenth century.[15] In fact, as Micheline R. Ishay and others have argued, this distinction reveals a historically parochial view of human history; in fact, ESC rights—as laws—can indeed be found in any number of formal law codes from cultures and religions around the world going back centuries and even millennia.[16] This is extremely important to remember as we think about faith-based intersections with human needs that reflect long-standing ethical and religious traditions.

Yet the concept of human rights goes far beyond the letter of the law. In social justice and humanitarian aid settings, allusions to rights often point to a moral concept, deeply rooted in ethical, humanitarian, and religious beliefs. In this view, rights are about existential entitlement—what we think people are entitled to simply on the basis of their identity as human beings, on moral commonalities that cross and go beyond religious traditions. In this way, the idea of rights becomes a moral tool for the realization of social justice, that is, how we work to provide what is due to human beings who suffer from the lack of bare necessities, from

disease, and from the wrongful behaviors of others. While philosophers continue to debate over the intellectual and moral foundations that would support and justify such views, persons of faith
who are engaged in everyday practical social justice efforts need
not choose between rights as laws and rights as moral or ethical entitlements rooted in identity issues related to beliefs about
God. Nor do they need—necessarily—to choose between rights
and "charitable" gifts, "agape love," hospitality, and civic duty. It
seems to me that the world and human need is big enough for all
of these to operate across relationships in an integrated manner
culturally suited within each particular society. Global health and
justice needs a multidisciplinary range of integrated models that
work—and that are used well. Let's look at how we got to modern
international rights related to health by starting with the history
of the Universal Declaration of Human Rights.

A SHORT HISTORY OF THE UDHR

The full history of the UDHR has been written by other scholars, among them Mary Ann Glendon and Johannes Morsink.[17]
Neither Glendon nor Morsink, however, explores in any great
detail how religious views influenced its creation, or how religious
debates shape the way it is viewed by faith-based organizations
doing social justice today.

The essential history of the UDHR begins with the United
Nations (UN). The UN was founded as part of a commitment
by American and British political powers to create a lasting
and peaceful solution to the problems that arose during and as
a result of World War Two. UN history begins in 1941, when
on June 12 in London various international powers signed the
"Inter-Allied Declaration," a commitment to "work together with
other free peoples, both in war and in peace."[18] This was followed
two months later by the Atlantic Charter, a proposal for certain principles for international collaboration to maintain peace

and security. The Charter was signed by US President Franklin Delano Roosevelt and the prime minister of the United Kingdom, Winston Churchill. Addressing Congress in Washington, DC, in 1941, Roosevelt summarized the vision behind these activities as, in his words, a world founded by four essential freedoms.[19] That is, Roosevelt argued, the efforts for peace and for the structures that would eventually lead to the UN came out of a united commitment to protect and ensure, "everywhere in the world," the (1) freedom of speech and expression, (2) freedom of worship, (3) freedom from want, and (4) freedom from fear.

In January 1942, amidst a world deep into war, twenty-six allied nations who were fighting together against the forces of Nazi Germany (as well as Japan after Pearl Harbor in December 1941) pledged support for the Atlantic Charter by signing a "Declaration by United Nations." Various conferences during the war then refined the agreements and brought in other countries as UN members, including, among others, China and the USSR. The UN was formally created six months after the end of World War Two, on October 24, 1945, the date when its charter was ratified. Its first big meeting, the first UN General Assembly, took place in London, in January 1946, and brought together representatives of fifty-one nations.[20] Related to this post-war global action on governing human rights across borders were decisions to create global economic bodies such as the World Bank.[21]

Thus the founding ideas for the UN took shape early in its history, before most nations or their leaders knew of the terrible atrocities that were taking place in Nazi-occupied territories. By 1946, as the fact of the Holocaust became increasingly well documented and recognized, citizens around the world reeled at its details, scale, and long-term implications for the need to create preventive international laws about human rights to ensure that such atrocities "never happen again." Even into the late 1960s and early 1970s, "never again" was the message that many American schoolchildren learned as a fundamental moral to frame world history. In my secular grade school and high school, I remember, this appeal to "never again" permeated just about everything we learned, and was fundamental in the underlying social ideals of my teachers and my classmates' older siblings, as they responded to the late 1960s' movement calling for lives marked by a serious commitment to political and social justice.

To prevent another war and another Holocaust, the UN was eager to establish laws that would have power across national borders. Thus one of the first goals of the new United Nations in 1945 was to create a common standard for international human rights. It was up to the UN's Commission on Human Rights, led by Eleanor Roosevelt (1884–1962, see full-page image at the beginning of this chapter), to bring this standard into being. As part of the organization of the United Nations, diplomats also initiated action that led to creation of a comparable global health organization, the World Health Organization (WHO), which came into force, like the UDHR, in 1948.

The UN Commission on Human Rights was made up of eighteen representatives. They came from Australia, Belgium, Byelorussia (today better known as Belarus), Chile, China, Egypt, France, India, Iran, Lebanon, Panama, the Philippines, Ukraine, the UK, the US, Uruguay, the USSR, and Yugoslavia. Representatives held a broad diversity of religious and philosophical beliefs (and non-beliefs).

For example, John Humphrey, the Canadian lawyer who wrote the first draft of the UDHR, drew on a commissioned report, from the newly formed United Nations Educational, Scientific and Cultural Organization (UNESCO), on human rights views and their foundations in ethical and legal standards around the world.[22] While Humphrey himself was an agnostic,[23] he worked closely on the final text with René Cassin. The French jurist who most influenced the final document, Cassin was a Jew who had lost most of his extended family to the Holocaust; Cassin was awarded the Nobel Peace Prize in 1968 for his role in the UDHR.[24]

The UDHR was also profoundly shaped by Peng-Chun Chang, a philosopher from China who was a scholar on Chinese and Buddhist thought, and Charles Malik, a devout Lebanese Christian philosopher who taught in a setting of Francophone Islam and Christian Orthodoxy. In contrast with Cassin's support for Israel, Malik was a spokesman for the Arab League.[25] Another central personality shaping ideas for the Declaration was Jacques Maritain, a Catholic and French Thomist philosopher.[26]

Not surprisingly, Commission meetings were lively. When it came to ESC rights, Humphrey later noted, "the two special interests that have tried hardest to influence the Declaration are the Catholic Church and the Communist Party—the former with considerably more success than the latter."[27] This was not meant as praise. In fact, Humphrey was critical of an underlying agenda, as Humphrey saw it, in which Catholic Social Teaching was, he felt, being used to hammer out certain views on women's work that he found counterproductive to the goal for a document marked by a language of equality. Humphrey was committed to maintaining objectivity about religious views in the UDHR. During the shaping of ESC rights on women and children in November 1948, for example, he wrote, "I dislike . . . the Roman Catholic campaign to write a particular philosophy into the Declaration."[28]

Nonetheless, Humphrey was not entirely unsympathetic to Christian ideals as he heard them from Catholic clergy. On a holiday to Brittany in September 1948, for example, reflecting on a sermon he had just heard, he wrote later in his diary:

> [The priest's message was essentially that] there is something, which we have learned to call the Christian ethic . . . without which life is mean and egotistical. It is mainly because . . . man has forgotten this ethic that the world has gotten itself into its present mess. I profoundly believe that this is true. . . . And this moral bankruptcy is the reason for our failure to organize peace. I once thought that socialism could fill this moral gap. . . . What we need is something like the Christian morality without the tommyrot.[29]

As a document enshrining international human rights, the UDHR was intended to be a first step only. It was intentionally designed as a "declaration," that is, containing no formal legal power that any of the countries who sign onto it would be obligated to enforce. It was hard enough to get nations to agree about the way they phrased the ideals. And yet the UDHR was seen as key to what would eventually become international law. It was meant to be part of an "International Bill of Rights," paired with a legal document, an "International Covenant," which ultimately took shape as two distinctly separate covenants, discussed further below.

Against this broad historical background, let's turn now to look more closely at how the UDHR relates to faith-based responses for the poor as they may advance a vision and realization of global health. In particular, let's examine the way that one article in the document—Article 25—relates to religious ideals about the provision of basic human needs, and how this religious perspective relates to ESC rights.

UDHR ARTICLE 25: WHAT IT IS AND HOW IT GOT THERE

As serious moral mandates, the essential elements of ESC rights are found in the Christian tradition in the parable of the sheep and goats in Matthew 25:31–46. This parable is across history perhaps the most frequently cited text for a faith-based response to poverty rooted in the justice of heaven. In this text, we find the "righteous"—those blessed by God and heirs of eternity—defined as people who feed the hungry, give water to the thirsty, welcome strangers, clothe the naked, provide medical care to the sick, and visit those in prison. These actions (later expanded to include burial of the dead, not mentioned in Matthew 25) are in the Catholic tradition called the "corporal works of mercy." And yet there is not one word about mercy in this particular biblical text. These behaviors, rather, are acts of *righteousness*, intended as physical activities meant to be enacted in a physical performance. There is nothing here of feelings, motives, or even charity; they are, rather simply actions based in what, Jesus says, God considers *right*. This cannot be emphasized enough. For it is in fact these very same essential *actions* that also shape UDHR Article 25, despite the fact that some conservative groups regard human rights arguments as oppositional to Christian ideals. In fact, even if it is a document that is nonsectarian and not (technically) binding by law, UDHR Article 25 has rather a lot in common with Matthew 25.

UDHR Article 25 is also a key foundational text in the contemporary global concern for health as a human right. While not everyone engaged in health justice for the poor will care about the religious expressions of the Christian tradition, UDHR Article 25 can serve as an essential "pier"—those supports in the middle of bridges that give them extra strength—to connect arms in common activities as they seek to work together for health and justice across the "God gap." The rest of this chapter will consider these seven behaviors through their codification in the establishment of this formative modern document and this particular UDHR Article.

UDHR Article 25 has two parts. The first part (25.1) is where we find the seven actions that are also mentioned in Matthew 25. This first part is a general statement about these rights in the wording as finally agreed upon by the United Nations Human Rights Commission whose job it was to create the Declaration. The second part (25.2) is a statement about special needs related to childbearing and childhood; 25.2 was originally a completely separate Article, merged here later—before the December 1948 vote on the final UDHR wording—because the Commission wanted to keep the UDHR as brief and concise as possible.[30] In its final version, Article 25 says:

(1) Everyone has the right to a standard of living adequate for the health and well-being of himself and his family, including food, clothing, housing and medical care and necessary social services, and the right to security in the event of unemployment, sickness, disability, widowhood, old age or other lack of livelihood in circumstances beyond his control.[31]

(2) Motherhood and childhood are entitled to special care and assistance. All children, whether born in or out of wedlock, shall enjoy the same social protection.

The concern expressed in Article 25.2 was particularly important in the context of social services in 1948. Just days before the final vote, the UNICEF chairman had described to the Commission how only 6 percent of the devastated population in post-war Europe was receiving the aid that it needed, that children made up one-third of this population, in addition to a large proportion of pregnant and breastfeeding mothers, and that the aid gap was creating an "abnormally high" level of infant mortality.[32]

To understand Article 25, we must begin with its immediate context in the UDHR as a whole. It is placed in the middle of the second half of the document, within the group that includes related Articles about social life and basic survival, Articles 22 through 28. These seven Articles define what are usually understood today as ESC rights. They affirm that "everyone as a member of society has the right" to "social security" and governmental protection of "the economic, social and cultural rights, indispensable for his dignity and the free development of his personality" (Article 22); work, free choice of employment (Article 23); rest and leisure, with "reasonable limitation of working hours and periodic holidays with pay" (Article 24); education, including "free" and "compulsory" elementary education, available technical and professional education, and merit-based access to higher education (Article 26); participation in community cultural life, the arts, and benefits of scientific advances (Article 27); and finally, a social and international order in which one can realize these rights and freedoms (Article 28).

Significantly, all of these ESC rights are closely interconnected with health. Health depends, that is, on the working conditions of a person and her or his family. Health depends on proper rest. Health choices depend on education, which shapes employment choices and economic resources. Health depends on one's ability to enjoy culture, arts, and scientific advances. And health is influenced by one's larger social community and national and international order. For example, children's greatest health risks are direct results of failures in these seven areas. Children are more likely to have poor health and grow up (if they grow up) to be poor adults with suboptimal health if they live in places marked by violence, unsafe housing, parents and neighbors who are struggling to survive, inadequate nutrition, deficient and unsafe schools, and lack of prompt and effective access to proper medical care and technological benefits simply because they are poor. These cultural or living-condition-related factors that affect wellness are known as the *social determinants of health*, defined and briefly discussed in Chapter 1. Effective global health depends on fixing these community and social problems at least as much as it depends on individual body-centered medicine. This is why ESC rights matter so much for faith-based communities who care about health and justice. Those in ministry are often working to help others in exactly these areas of need simply as a part of their routine spiritual and pastoral care, wherever they live. But let's get back to Article 25 and look at its broader legal context, as part of the UDHR document as a whole.

Johannes Morsink has described in detail how Article 25 took shape.[33] Its central core was the assertion of a universal right of the human person to "security in the event of unemployment, sickness, disability, widowhood, old age, or other lack of livelihood in circumstances beyond his control." Article 25 is the only place in the UDHR where health-care rights are spelled out, to include food, clothing, housing, and medical care.

As noted earlier, the debates over Article 25 also led to extensive discussion about ESC rights as something "new" compared to "old" civil and political rights. Overall, the UDHR Committee insisted that both ESC and civil and political rights were equally important, and Committee members fought against what they felt to be an artificial distinction.[34] The distinction between moral/ethical and legal rights was also understood in different ways by different country members of the Committee, depending in part on their culture as well as their personal and religious beliefs. Even today there are secular scholars who may affirm ESC rights as international law but who nevertheless doubt their philosophical claim to any universal basis in moral "truth." According to some opinions, the power and appeal of the public human rights rhetoric has moved beyond a defensible dialectic to border on the creation of a secular religion.[35]

In any case, the struggle to keep ESC and civil and political rights together within an International Bill of Rights ultimately failed. When the long-promised covenant on human rights was finally adopted and open for signature in 1966, it was—for logistical and administrative reasons—split into two separate covenants, the International Covenant on Civil and Political Rights (ICCPR) and the International Covenant on Economic, Social and Cultural Rights (ICESCR). The tragedy of this split is that States that sign off on one of these two documents have no obligation to sign off on the other; the United States, for example, has ratified (agreed to treat as legally binding legislation within its national borders) the ICCPR, but it has not ratified the ICESCR.[36]

A brief glimpse at how the committee chose various details helps to illustrate how very human—and global—the creation of the UDHR was. In shaping Article 25, Humphrey drew on constitutions around the world where the four fundamental material needs also listed in Matthew 25—food, clothing, shelter, and medical care—were in fact included in what was viewed as "everyone's minimum reasonable demands upon the rest of humanity."[37] Even so, the Commission almost cut these phrases out of the final document to keep it short. Happily, delegates from the USSR and China objected, and so these four specifics remain in the document. The Chilean delegation proposed that the article be more explicit about the importance of public health and safety, and Humphrey himself prefaced this affirmation with the sentence, "Everyone has the right to medical care."[38] The right to medical care was in accord with virtually all constitutions of member delegates (with the obvious exception of the United States[39]). Yugoslavia and most Latin American nations had constitutions that gave citizens a right to cheap and sanitary housing. And the American Law Institute, together with Panama and Cuba, had drafted and affirmed the universal right to adequate food and housing. Only the right to food was "a novel addition."[40] Yet even such basic rights as these four left a lot of wiggle room for different countries. Food and medical needs may be fairly consistent across the human condition, but adequate clothing and housing depend, of course, on climate and local environment.

Legal concepts often affected debates over wording in the UDHR, since, after all, it was written to serve as a foundation that would help enshrine moral agreements into the force of (later) law. A legal right must, by definition, be something that can take place reasonably and realistically in real time or there is no point in making it a law. For example, I may believe I have a right to *be healthy*, but no human service or government can absolutely guarantee an ideal such as *health*. Furthermore, a legal right must be clear enough that nations that have agreed to be held accountable to UN standards can be judged, yet it must also be one that people in low- and middle-income countries can enjoy. These concerns shaped the final wording in Article 25 on the right to health. Humphrey wanted it to affirm a "right to medical care," but Eleanor Roosevelt, as head of the Commission, intervened. The result, adopted from the World Health Organization Constitution, affirms a universal right to "the highest attainable standard of health." Since health is a result of social and physical determinants and behaviors, Article 25 essentially packages together key ingredients in these health determinants, leaving it to the ICESCR (discussed further below) and other formal legal treaties to define what legal realization of health and health-care services will look like.

To be universal, rights must also apply to all persons, regardless of their nation's resource limitations; a food shortage in a particular country must never deny the individuals of that country their universal human *right* to food, nor should it ever give the rest of the world an excuse to let them starve. This emphasis in the UDHR's affirmation means, for example, that a sick orphan in a very poor and unstable nation has the same right to food, housing, and health that I have in the rich West; the global logistical challenge is of course to ensure that proper and just redistribution of resources to truly address her needs actually takes place in real time and without injustice to others. By keeping to a language of rights as universal and absolute, the UDHR serves as a reminder that international cooperation (or neglect) can profoundly affect cross-border resources—and risks.

The inclusion of the terms "food and clothing" and "social security" in UDHR Article 25 was also subject to lively debate. Persuasively defending the inclusion of "food and clothing," the Chinese delegate P. C. Chang drew on Confucian ideals of benevolence to note that he "did not see what possible objection there could be to that phrase when millions of people throughout the world were deprived of food and clothing."[41] Alexei Pavlov, the USSR delegate, fought hard for more specific wording on housing and medical assistance. He lost, but the Article subcommittee added a reference to rights to "social security" and a "standard of living."

The phrase "social security" turned out to be quite controversial, and not because it was quickly becoming the catchphrase for FDR's national plan in America. All committee members concurred that the phrase "social security" explicitly implied some level of public state-ordered assurance of the social resources necessary to ensure basic material needs. The challenge was how to phrase it in a way that everyone could agree on.

To us today, after the final vote and with nearly seventy years of living with the resulting document, the whole debate over whether to say "social security" in Article 25 might seem odd, since we can easily glance up the document itself and see that Article 22 says quite clearly that "everyone as a member of society, has the right to social security." But, in fact, Article 22 was finalized by the Committee after Article 25, and the phrase "social security" was included in Article 22 because of a now-inexplicable misperception about what the Committee agreed on in their preliminary votes about wording for Article 25. Anxious that the phrase not be omitted entirely, several delegates—led by René Cassin—insisted on adding it to Article 22, which is a general summary of ESC rights. Efforts to smooth out the two references by substituting other phrases ultimately failed.[42] The final version of Article 25 was intended to affirm a right to "social security in the event of unemployment, sickness, [etc.]" but by a simple clerical error, the word "social" got left out, and thus the final text of the UDHR—faithful to its voters' hard-wrought decisions—even today retains the traces of these human inconsistencies. The fact that the drafters were content to leave both Articles untouched in the final vote, even after realizing what had happened, is a testimony to how important the concept of social security was to their vision of universal human economic and social rights.

On December 10, 1948, the UDHR as a completed document was voted into existence for use around the world by all UN member States. Its nature as a nonbinding declaration—one that "floats above all local and regional contingencies and is a statement of more or less abstract moral rights and principles"[43]— helped its rapid acceptance and recognition. Yet in fact it was to have immense international influence. Humphrey went so far as to argue in his memoirs that it became "part of the customary law of nations."[44] In the late 1990s, a survey by the legal historian Hurst Hannum showed how the UDHR has shaped dozens of international documents that do have real legal power to address what UDHR founders called the "moral gap."[45]

WHY RELIGION IS NOT MENTIONED IN THE UDHR

The controversies about how to describe exactly why, philosophically, the statements in the UDHR represented such broadly accepted global ideals were heated from the start. It was this debate more than anything else that kept explicit language about God out of the final document, despite the strong religious loyalties of many of its creators. Charles Malik, for example, originally wanted the UDHR to include a reference to God, making God the "guarantor of natural law, which judges all man-made law."[46] He was overruled, on the objection that the UDHR was meant for the world, including persons who had no religious beliefs and/or would not be able to agree with such a statement. The Brazilian delegations proposed similar amendments, linking reason and conscience with "creation in the image and likeness of God" and human dignity founded on "man's divine origin and immortal destiny."[47] Both suggestions died when it became clear how strongly others objected. To do any good, they agreed, the UDHR must first be something nations are willing to agree with, even in principle. The basic moral truths it contained did not require everyone to agree on *why* they mattered. Even the phrase "by nature" was fraught with debate over "metaphysical problems."[48] As the Polish delegate cautioned, the UDHR was "a United Nations document which could not properly deal with metaphysical questions."[49] The result—or at least the intended result—was that anyone could affirm the UDHR, whatever her or his views on religion, without any qualms over compromise, and without needing to conform to any single perspective on why one believed these rights to be valid for all human persons. The role of human nature and the idea of "natural rights" continued to influence many UDHR authors in the years that followed. Although this debate over God language was central to the committee's work on Article 1 rather than Article 25, it reminds us that faith was immensely important to many members in defining practical activities related to human rights for health.

FROM DECLARATION TO COVENANT(S)

The UDHR still today explicitly and directly influences interpretation of ESC rights in actual law, through its role in the two Covenants that were to follow, the International Covenant on Civil and Political Rights (ICCPR) and the International Covenant on Economic, Social and Cultural Rights (ICESCR). Indeed, all three documents today make up the UN's International Bill of Rights. Work on the two Covenants started as soon as the UDHR was final, but proceeded at a glacial pace for many years. It was not until 1966 that the two Covenants were finally adopted and ready for ratification. And it was another full decade before they actually "entered into force" or became legally enforceable documents in international law, ICESCR first, on January 3, 1976, and the ICCPR soon afterward, on March 23, 1976.[50]

The content of the two Covenants is integrally linked to the UDHR Articles. Each Covenant addresses the relevant claims in the UDHR and spells out what this means for legal implementation. The ideas in UDHR Article 25 are the subject of ICESCR Articles 9 through 12. For instance, Article 11 is about the right to food, clothing, and housing. It mandates, for example, "an equitable distribution of world food supplies in relation to need" in a manner that considers "the problems of both food-importing and food-exporting countries."[51] International law on the right to health is found in ICESCR Article 12. This Article mandates that steps be taken to: improve infant survival and development;

improve environmental and industrial hygiene; prevent, treat, and control all disease; and "the creation of conditions which would assure to all medical services and medical attention in the event of sickness" (ICESCR 12d).

Many other legal and advisory documents have followed over the years, based on these three key sources. For each of the rights enshrined in the two Covenants, the respective UN Committee has also issued documents known as "General Comments." General Comments serve to interpret these standards as they affect countries' obligations to ensure that people's rights are realized in practice.[52] The right to health (ICESCR Article 12) is interpreted in the United Nations' Committee on Social and Cultural Rights (CSCR) General Comment 14. General Comment documents are important because they serve as official guideposts for how member States ought to interpret and apply each of the different rights. In addition, neutral official spokespersons who have international renown for their expertise in various areas serve term UN appointments as "special rapporteurs" on particular rights. For example, two of the "special rapporteurs," one on the Right to Health and another on the Right to Food, have issued occasional statements also intended to help clarify and expand human rights activities for those who suffer violations of these rights.[53]

A number of other legal documents have also emerged from regional organizations or from a focus on a population subset or group. Such documents include, for example, the European Convention on Human Rights (1950);[54] The African Charter on Human and Peoples' Rights (1981);[55] and the African Charter on the Rights and Welfare of the Child (1990).[56] Other major legal conventions that also have international relevance include the Convention against Torture and Other Cruel, Inhuman or Degrading Treatment or Punishment (1984);[57] the International Convention on the Elimination of all Forms of Racial Discrimination (1965);[58] the Convention on the Rights of the Child (CRC) (1989);[59] the Convention on the Rights of Persons with Disabilities (2006);[60] and the International Convention on the Elimination of All Forms of Discrimination Against Women (CEDAW) (1979).[61] Each of these contains protective aspects relevant to health-related issues.

These documents are legally binding in international law to States that choose to sign them into law for their respective countries. Beyond these legally binding documents, there are many other nonbinding statements and declarations (like the UDHR itself). The fame and weight that these various documents have to influence international dialogue about human rights varies widely. Since my focus in this chapter is on a basic and concise summary of the story of UDHR Article 25, these other documents will not be discussed here.

FAITH IN THE FIELD: BUILDING A VISION FOR HOPE

While faith-based relief and aid activities may focus on individuals and families in the private sector of a community, positive results that last often require buy-in or changes at the level of those who make and enforce rules, standards, and laws. As emphasized in other chapters, global health is about multidisciplinary integration. The better equipped one is with a range of tools, the richer and more potentially healing the conversations may be for good. Sometimes all it takes to open a door for opportunity is to speak truth kindly: to identify that a particular violence is a rights violation. To name what is wrong—with a realistic and wise hope—can perhaps create one step toward imagining a better world and, possibly, empowering that vision toward action.

When it comes to human rights, this "power to name" is important because many of the people in positions for such conversations around the world are people of religious faith. Engaging with the poor in an understanding of the documents of their own faith can also help foster collaborative trust that strengthens the goals that underlie ESC rights. For example, two scholars with the Tufts University Feinstein International Center had this experience:

> One large agency operation in Afghanistan today realized that most of its local Afghan employees had only a very rudimentary knowledge of their religion, coming as they did from remote rural settings. The aid agency helped find an Imam who would come into their office and offer classes on the Koran and spiritual guidance for those who wished to attend. Attendance was high and the agency reports that workers [sic] commitment to the mission of the agency seemed to grow. We should note that this was an avowedly Christian agency.[62]

Human rights documents have limitations. For example, they cannot create or ensure justice simply because they exist, or because we know about them. They are tools that can best be used in combination with other resources. Yet clearly one of the first steps in preventing the abuse and violation of other human beings is simply to know what comprises injustice. A faith-based group or individual who is able to speak intelligently about even the most basic concept of entitlements and rights can send a strong message of value for human dignity and capacity building. Educating people about basic rights—as a universal moral concept that is also protected by international law—is not a cure-all for the world's problems. But it can encourage people to work for changes that they now only dream about. Religious volunteers or missionaries who choose *not* to talk about—and work for—human rights (or act as if they do not matter or are against their religious beliefs) may undermine their own desire to be good agents for community, individual, or world healing. They may also lose the credibility of those they work with, offering as charity what texts in their own religious tradition—such as Matthew 25—define as mandated acts of righteousness. Faith-based charity in health care (discussed further in Chapter 6), if it denies or ignores human rights, risks seriously failing to address the real system issues that cause disease, even as it also alienates potential colleagues in medical and public health. In fact, there is no reason for Christians to shy away from talking about human rights in social justice and health care for the poor. Tools for social and economic justice are just that: tools. They may work most effectively when they are used not in oppositional ways, but rather in concert—each tool honed and used to address what it is best designed to do. A very large proportion of influential Christian leaders—present and past, including those of both conservative and liberal persuasion—affirm that "rights talk" is in fact both relevant and compatible with the Christian tradition.

Bas de Gaay Fortman is perhaps one of the most encouraging modern voices on religion in ESC rights today. Fortman is a Dutch Christian Protestant diplomat and scholar based at Utrecht, who lived through World War Two as a child in the Netherlands (where his grandmother died of starvation during the "Dutch Hunger Winter" of 1944–1945).[63] "Although . . . [f]aith-based approaches to human rights cannot be of universal character," Fortman notes,

> these distinct perspectives do not necessarily affect the universal nature of human rights as such. At the same time, such linking to the sources of faith in the equal dignity and worth of wo/men and their inherent freedoms and responsibilities may play a vital part in establishing a genuine global human rights constituency.[64]

Fortman also draws on the 1992 Latin American bishops' endorsement of human rights to emphasize how much human rights concepts have in common with the three Abrahamic religions.[65] He points explicitly to the biblical idea of *tzedakah,* a word that has the same meaning in its Hebrew, Christian Syriac, and Arabic cognates. Often translated as "charity" or alms," the fundamental meaning of tzedakah is "righteousness"; languages that use this word implicitly therefore link these two ideas as a single inseparable concept. Thus, as Fortman puts it, "the connection with religion may provide the necessary cultural basis for the struggle for economic, social and cultural rights."[66]

The justice of ESC rights was further affirmed in the 2008 Russian Orthodox Bishops' Council on human dignity, freedom, and rights. In summary, the Orthodox Church, said the bishops,

> stresses the legitimacy of property rights, the right to work, the protection from employers' malpractices, but also the legitimacy of the right of free entrepreneurship, as well as the right to a decent quality of life. Yet the stipulation that these rights are legitimate is to keep their 'moral dimension' central, and hence to assert the inferiority of rights to religious goals. The crucial issue of these rights is 'to prevent confrontation and disparity in society.'[67]

Not everyone in the Orthodox Church today agrees with this view, just as not every Christian philosopher or ethicist agrees that it is possible to have a meaningful conversation about human rights or "natural law" between people of faith and people with secular views of human rights that do not include concepts of the divine. My point here is not to argue that there be some uniform agreement, but rather to point to the value of such cross-disciplinary and religious-secular conversations in the context of humanitarian aid and social justice activities relevant to global health efforts.

EARLY CHRISTIAN VOICES ON HUMAN RIGHTS

A statement like that of the Russian Orthodox Bishops' Council reminds us that modern human rights are viewed seriously even by those we may think of as religious traditionalists. While many ecumenical Christian groups embrace human rights ideas easily, health-care initiatives around the world often depend on groups that have both a strong commitment to the poor and a strong commitment to a more theologically "conservative" viewpoint, often one that holds to or values the authority of early Christian sources as serious models for faith and life. Indeed, human rights as they relate to economic and social poverties are not just for liberals any more than they are limited to post-Enlightenment values. They are deeply interwoven into views on social justice that go way back to concepts that we find in sources from late antiquity. It is in these contexts that we must especially keep in mind that "rights" mean more than their legal definition in a this-world court of law.

Among conservative Christian views that dismiss rights talk as irrelevant—or so relative as to be meaningless—the most famous (or perhaps infamous) is that which has been much quoted from Alasdair MacIntyre's 1981 *After Virtue,* where he noted that "Natural or human rights are fictions . . . There are no such rights, and belief in them is one with belief in witches and unicorns."[68] While MacIntyre's comment is only a small part of a deeply nuanced moral philosophy that reaches far beyond our discussion here, a number of serious Christian ethicists, philosophers, and theologians have refuted this particular statement of MacIntyre's at length.[69] Yale philosopher Nicholas Wolterstorff, for example, calls MacIntyre's positioning "an attack on a straw man."[70] And Catholic historian Roger Ruston, who has worked on human rights language in sixteenth-century Dominican preaching, argues that "Despite the significance given by MacIntyre to moral traditions, his arguments do not pay much attention to actual history."[71] Whatever our view on MacIntyre's broader philosophy, his view on natural rights—at least as it is encapsulated in this memorable *koan*—does not in fact appear to reflect the views found in many of the most formative historical texts about ESC rights in Christian tradition.

While Nicholas Wolterstorff is sometimes associated with the evangelical "right," he in fact offers the most explicit modern recognition of human rights language in pre-Enlightenment Christian tradition. For example, remembering an experience in

South Africa in 1976 that was very similar to Daniel Cohen's "aha moment" with Mustafa Barghouti, Wolterstorff said that:

> As to the claim one often hears that the idea of rights is alien to Christianity, that the idea was invented by secular thinkers of the Enlightenment . . . I say, to the contrary, that recent scholarship makes it indisputably clear that the idea of natural rights was explicitly and prolifically employed by the canon lawyers of the 1100s and again by leaders in the early Reformed tradition.[72]

In fact, Wolterstorff emphasizes, we find human rights in even more ancient texts, including patristic texts from late antiquity. In his book *Justice: Rights and Wrongs*, citing John Chrysostom's sermons on wealth and poverty at length while also pointing to similar themes in Ambrose and Basil of Caesarea, he concludes:

> I see no other way to interpret what John [Chrysostom] is doing with his powerful rhetoric than that he is reminding his audience, rich and poor alike, of the *natural rights* of the poor. . . . The recognition of natural rights is unmistakably there: The poor are wronged because they do not have what is theirs by natural right, what they have a natural right to.[73]

Indeed, most patristic texts about the poor in fact echo some of the same economic and social concerns that we find in UDHR Article 25. Both share a sense of imperative: that the needy *must rightly* receive food equity, health care, fair access to drinking water, debt resolution and relief, fair employment practices, preservation of family inheritance related to property, and adequate housing. Patristic authors differ from the Commission on Human Rights, of course, by talking quite a lot about God—and they often have underlying assumptions about social status, patronage, and position that may run counter to modern views on democracy and equality. And yet they share the UDHR focus that aid must be rooted in the nature of reality, including the reality of the human person and human condition. And as Wolterstorff observes, even John Chrysostom—more commonly viewed as a supporter of benevolent patronage rather than human rights of the poor—presents human need and accountability to the needy in terms that remarkably resemble UDHR Article 25.

One way that patristic texts go beyond the UDHR is that they are clearer about *obligations*. To help the poor is, according to some early Christian texts, the obligation of anyone who has more than what he or she needs for basic subsistence. Even patristic authors such as Clement of Alexandria, for example, who defend the Christian's freedom to own, keep, and even store up private property, are uncompromising in their insistence of moral obligations to provide concrete material substances to those who lack.[74]

One of the most explicit patristic texts on human rights is perhaps that of Gregory of Nazianzus, in his *Oration* 14, a sermon on homeless and diseased beggars, written sometime between 368 and 380 CE. Gregory calls for Christians to imitate the *isotes*, that is, equality or evenhandedness of God; one translator renders it "the justice of God."[75] Gregory also used the word *isonomia*, a Greek political term that could mean either "equity" or "equality of rights" in the legal sense (*nomos*). Appealing to the Garden of Eden before the Fall, Gregory says, "I would have you look back to our primary equality of rights [*isonomia*], not the later diversity. . . . As far as you can, support nature, honor primeval liberty, show reverence for yourself, . . . help to resist sickness, offer relief to human need." (Or. 14.26) Other Greek-speaking authors contemporary with Gregory also defined the human persons as having equal worth, at least before God, and roundly condemned inequities. Asterius of Amasea, for example, regarded material inequality (he calls it *anomalia*, from which we get *anomaly*) as innately unjust. Covetousness, he says, creates a "marked disparity in the conditions of life between human persons created equal in worth."[76]

And the writings of Basil of Caesarea, while they do not speak of rights, do also insist on civic justice rooted in material equity and a created order in which God shares the world generously with everyone.[77]

RIGHTS AND PIETY: LACTANTIUS ON JUSTICE AND WORSHIP

Lactantius (c. 250–c.325 CE) is another patristic author who deserves far more attention than he has received to date for his concern with human rights and social justice. A Latin convert to Christianity who moved from Carthage in North Africa to northwest Asia Minor (near modern Istanbul) in the late third century, Lactantius discusses social justice, including a reference to rights, at length in his *Divine Institutes*, particularly in Book 5 (on justice) and Book 6 (on "true worship").[78] His arrival in Asia Minor as a Christian coincided with the emperor Diocletian's "Great Persecution" and may be the reason that he quickly moved west, eventually appointed tutor to Crispus, son of the emperor Constantine around 310; Book 5 of the *Divine Institutes* opens with an address to Constantine. While Lactantius himself was among the educated elite in his society, as a Christian he knew all too well the social, fiscal, and material insecurities that went along with choosing Christ in an era of political opposition.

Lactantius emphasizes the fundamental social equity inherent in true justice. Indeed, he claims, justice is at heart an inseparable coherence of *piety* and *equity* (or "fairness").[79] As all human persons are created by God, he says, "no one is cut off from God's celestial benevolence. Just as God divides his unique light equally between all, makes springs flow, supplies food," and sleep, Lactantius says, so, too, "No one is a slave with him and no one is a master, for if 'he is the same father to everyone,' so are we all his children with *equal rights*."[80] In fact, he reiterates, "the whole force of justice lies in the fact that everyone who comes into this human estate on equal terms is made equal by it."[81] He argues, in a manner that might seem radical, that Christians do not differentiate between rich and poor or free and slave; riches, he says, "cause no distinction except for their power to make people notable for good works . . . for acts of justice."[82] For the Latin jurists, such as Lactantius's near-contemporary, the third-century Roman jurist Ulpian, justice (*iustitia*) was "a steady and enduring will to render to each their right or desert"; and *ius* can also mean "right."[83]

In Book 6, on "true worship," Lactantius moves on to define and expand on the central role of justice. To act justly toward God is, he says, called religion; to act justly toward other human beings is "compassion or humanity."[84] Here indeed we find ourselves outside the framework of rights as entitlements codified in civic law, where, instead, "rights" and "justice" overlap with moral concepts identified with ideals of the heart. Yet Lactantius's arguments are, like such discussions in modern rights rhetoric, based in an assumption that the way we treat others in need is something due to them, as part of God's justice, and not some undeserved nicety that incidentally bubbles up out of our good moral intentions.

Giving resources to the poor, says Lactantius, must be indiscriminate:

> Why pick special people? Why check for looks? If someone prays to you because he thinks you are a human being, then you must treat him as a human being too . . . grab hold of true justice in its true form. Give to the blind, the sick, the lame, and the destitute. . . . Cherish them as much as you can, and sustain their souls with humanity. . . . Anyone who can help a dying man but doesn't is his murderer.[85]

Lactantius then goes on to define such justice further. It is not when we provide for friends, relatives, and commonly expected social obligations. Rather, true justice is when we provide for "the needy and the useless,"[86] with food, hospitality, ransom for captives, health care for the sick, and in burying strangers and paupers.

Clearly an optimist, Lactantius often offers advice that seems extreme. "A rich man with God can never be poor," he says. To anyone who might be afraid that this obligation to respond to news about some catastrophe or public crisis will wipe out their inheritance through this mandate to care for the needy, he says, do it anyway. A few lines later, however, he does soften his position a bit, with a realistic concession. "If you cannot manage great deeds on your own," he admits, "practice justice as best you can . . . switch to a better purpose what you were about to spend on rubbish."[87] Throughout the *Divine Institutes*, Lactantius emphasizes the traditional view that such behaviors, if they don't profit you visibly in this life, will win God's recognition and reward in the next. Yet this is more than simply redemptive almsgiving. His central focus affirms a linkage of redemption with *justice,* that is, equal rights and fundamental human entitlements of the poor to basic securities like food, clothing, housing, and health care.

Lactantius lived through an era when Christians suffered what we today would call violations of civil and political rights. To be a Christian, that is, invalidated any prior protected social status in the eyes of the law; one lost the right to any court appeal, since Christians were regarded as traitors to the state. They were subject to loss of property rights and in many cases life itself, often in a most gruesome manner. And yet even though he wrote the *Divine Institutes* during the years when Christianity was, under Constantine, gaining a new legal status, Lactantius's discussion of justice in these two books is not on ensuring or strengthening civil and political rights but instead on ESC rights—basic material rights for the poor and most socially vulnerable in society. He says of himself, in fact, "I never went into public life."[88] In other words, he taught rhetoric (a form of legal education in the ancient world) but never practiced as a lawyer or jurist.[89] Thus we can take his focus on ESC rights as support for the concern, throughout this chapter, on "rights" as a moral concept that might be implied in a codified Roman law but reaches much more broadly across faith-based ideals and actions.

And yet law codes in the late antique Christian era do in fact include some clear legal preoccupation with both civil and political, and ESC rights such as food for the starving. The Theodosian Code, a compilation of legal statements from the third to fifth centuries, contains at least a few rulings about food, clothing, and medical care for the poor, all from the Christian era. One early law of Constantine's enacted in 315 CE with revisions or amendments noted in 329, orders that, throughout Italy at least, "If any parent should report that he has offspring which on account of poverty he is not able to rear, there shall be no delay in issuing food and clothing, since the rearing of a newborn infant will not allow any delay."[90] Constantine here rules that aid must issue from state funds "without distinction." Another law, dated 322, addresses the problem of "provincials" (Roman citizens living in what is today North Africa) who out of poverty sell or pledge their children; here the emperor likewise rules that aid be issued "from the State storehouses. . . . For it is at variance with Our character that we should allow any person to be destroyed by hunger."[91] CT 13.3.8, dated to 368 and 370, legislates what translator Clyde Pharr called "socialized medicine." This law ordered the appointment of district physicians in Constantinople who, "knowing that their subsistence allowances are paid from the taxes of the people, shall prefer to minister to the poor honorably rather than to serve the rich shamefully."[92] The eighteenth-century physician Dr. Benjamin Rush, discussed in Chapter 1, might have agreed. Another law, dated to 416 and apparently targeting the city of Alexandria, ensured tax exemption for clergy who served as "attendants to the sick" (*parabolani*).[93] Those eligible for this particular office—their numbers are controlled and subject to public appointment—included "the

poor from the guilds, in proportion to the [city's] population."
Two years later this law was amended to increase the number of
permitted state-funded attendants, "who are assigned to care for
the suffering bodies of the sick . . . and . . .[are] experienced in
the practice of healing."[94]

Such laws addressed other economic concerns beyond that of
health care. A ruling dated to 443 suspended all debts and interest payments due from landowners in Africa who had lost their
property or fortunes as a result of the Vandal invasions. This law
explicitly noted its motivation as both "pity" as well as an appeal
to "the path of equity."[95] While laws about tax relief in times of crisis were fairly common in Roman antiquity, this is an interesting
conjunction of justice and mercy seen here in a legal statement.
The pairing of justice and mercy was of course also a standard
element in the ancient moral ideals found in Jewish law codified
in Hebrew scripture.[96]

I am not suggesting that global aid efforts today should
embrace an affirmation of Christian or late Roman law; this
would be a culturally inappropriate anachronism that could risk
advancing and perpetuating biases such as patronage, gender
discrimination, slavery, and torture, practices tolerated by early
Christians that we today condemn as destructive to social, mental, and physical health. Indeed, not all such laws from Roman
antiquity were kind to the poor. CT 14.18.1, dated 382, is the first
law in the Christian era against beggars. This law allows informers to report able-bodied beggars, who, if examined and found
to have no disability, would lose their civil liberties and could
be forced to serve their informers as slaves.[97] And while Gregory
of Nazianzus in his homily on the love of the poor (Oration
14) roundly condemned those who dismissively said the poor
deserved what they got in life, he and others also supported giving special help to those who fall suddenly into afflictions, suggesting a bias that favors aiding citizens from the upper class who
get into economic trouble over those who have suffered desperate
need much of their lives.

WE'RE ALL ON THE MAP

This chapter has explored how human rights is a central theme in economic and social justice related to poverty and health—the very areas where faith-based activists, medical workers, volunteers, and missionaries tend to work today. It argues against the idea that human rights are just something for liberals, something that can be reduced to post-Enlightenment "moral relativism." In fact, the idea of human rights has deep roots in history with strong strands of continuity in the way moral ideals argue social justice for those who are poor, hungry, dispossessed, and sick.

I am *not* saying ancient religious writers thought just as we do today; clearly there are many differences.[98] Despite these differences, however, those who currently work in social justice, activism, and health care initiatives with ties in the Christian tradition must be mindful that a solid subset of these historical faith-based texts do clearly mandate what even conservative writers discussed in this chapter have recognized as a "rights" claim to entitlement. Despite often profound philosophical differences, it frequently appears that those who work in secular and religious organizations have, in fact, much in common, including shared values for human rights that relate to food, clothing, shelter, and health care.

Just as ESC rights can support a shared space across the bridge between secular and religious activism, so, too, action for economic and social justice also intersects with concerns about civil and political rights. We see this in the early Christian Roman laws about state-funded health care for the very poor, as well as tax relief for the recently impoverished landowner. We see this in the historical role of "ordinary" religious believers who practiced nineteenth-century American public health as part of their civic duty, a theme explored in Chapter 3. And, too, we also see this intersection in contemporary encounters in poor communities around the world today. A closing story will illustrate why in fact

ESC rights as they relate to global health cannot be detached from or subordinated to civil and political rights.

Human rights lawyer Alicia Ely Yamin tells the story of an encounter she had in 1997 in Chiapas, southern Mexico, in a community marked by paramilitary violence.[99] The violence had erupted because of local poor villagers' concerns about the economic impact that the recently approved North American Free Trade Agreement (NAFTA) would have on their livelihood, on their economic survival. Those affected were mostly poor indigenous persons who hold to traditional Mayan beliefs and practices. These indigenous revolutionaries—called Zapatistas—used both force (especially when attacked) and increasing emphasis on non-violent resistance to oppose the Mexican state's political choices on trade. The economic uncertainties had quickly led to civil strife between those loyal to the government's support for NAFTA and those resisting such rule and its implications for their way of life.

Yamin was traveling through the area as part of a human rights contingent that was talking with those affected on both sides of the conflict. In one community during her visit, a village torn by divisive tensions, civil distrust, and violence, she met a woman who was hemorrhaging with a late-term miscarriage. In any society this condition is a medical emergency. Such a miscarriage inevitably means that one loses the child, whether the mother is treated or not; but treatment is vital to make sure the mother doesn't die, too. In Yamin's hometown in the United States, late miscarriage could be treated quickly, easily, and safely, with a few hours of outpatient care. It is emotionally devastating to lose a child wherever you live, but the point is that such a miscarriage—with proper health care—need not be dangerous to maternal health. In Chiapas, Yamin knew, there was a perfectly adequate public health facility near the woman's home that could provide the care she needed. And yet, she learned, the woman's family had chosen to do nothing, chosen to let her bleed to death at home, since in their view the health facility was "on the other side" in the conflict and so perceived as enemy territory. Better, they thought, to let her "die with dignity" than compromise the honor of the family and community by crossing over to the other side, to ask help from those responsible for massacres, disruption, and displacement in their village life.

Yamin was incensed. Here was a woman who had a basic human right to life and adequate medical care, whose rights were being violated by political and family choices. Her survival—or death—should not depend on such tensions when help was so close and available.

Her outrage was shaped by a deeper, more personal and recent sorrow. For she had come to Mexico that week on purpose in part to overcome a temptation to self-pity after she herself suffered a miscarriage at exactly the same stage in a pregnancy as this woman she sat with. "I dropped the neutral human rights investigator [role]," she remembers, "and I made sure that this woman was accompanied by an impartial NGO to the hospital and received the treatment that she needed and was returned to her community."

It was not random serendipity, Yamin recalls, emphatically, that this woman's life was at risk unnecessarily while she herself had received the best care in world-class health facilities just a few days earlier in New York City. It was not a case of "but for the grace of God" that she could act and be healed and this woman could not. Rather, she reminds us, "It was because of very human choices about laws and policies, about women's education and health facilities," about class and race.

As a result of this experience and others in her career, Yamin calls for scholars and activists alike to respond to such discrepancies and injustices by imagining other, better worlds, here and now. Yamin's work is known for its intellectual rigor. And yet, she insists, "This is not an intellectual thing; it's a visceral feeling about the outrageous arbitrariness." For, she reminds us,

> It is we who live in the Global North who are privileged, and
> our policy makers, our representatives, who need to understand

that we all live in the same world. We need to locate ourselves on the same political map. Because it is the decisions that are taken in Washington and London and at the G20 summits that determine the possibilities for enjoying health rights among the vast majority of people in the Global South as well as among the disadvantaged in this country.

Such visceral outrage is indeed the essence of much motivation to moral action around the world. Such outrage at the atrocities of World War Two shaped the broad appeal of the UDHR and its ability in 1948 to gain acceptance even by many who could not necessarily agree over why they agreed with it. A visceral commitment to faith-based moral choices may also inform, for many, the centuries-old appeal of the Matthew 25 parable. Feelings are not necessary for acting justly, of course, but they can certainly help energize inner resistance to apathy or burnout. "And that visceral feeling," Yamin concludes, "needs to lead us to act upon that manifest injustice. In applying a human rights framework to health, it makes us think about how we understand our own suffering and that of others."

In conclusion, this chapter has outlined the reasons that it is important for anyone active in faith-based responses to poverty to understand international legal history and concepts of economic, social, and cultural (ESC) rights, and be able to talk about them in an informed manner that will respect and foster dialogue with others in global health initiatives around the world (and in the United States) who may not share or sympathize with their religious views. The chapter provides a practical summary of Article 25 of the 1948 Universal Declaration of Human Rights (UDHR) and its relationship to religion and health. Though often contended or ignored, such documents possess real legal power that extends beyond the common laws and social norms of most countries that have either ignored or to various degrees consented to them. Through narrative examples from past and present history, the chapter outlines why most such documents say little about religion and yet in fact are crucial to all of us who live on the global map, intersecting health, religion, culture, art, and the desperation of injustice and human need.

Human rights–based approaches to health and social justice are not a magic bullet. As this chapter has shown (I hope), appeals to human rights raise a number of concerns and controversies. The nature of these concerns and controversies vary depending on how rights are understood, defined, and contextualized. Rights-based approaches to health—through litigation and legal enforcement—can often genuinely make a positive difference,[100] but they are just one part of a human response that respects and engages with those who are limited by the sufferings of poverty. As Rowan Williams, former archbishop of Canterbury, puts it, "the denial of rights is a terrible thing; and what takes time to learn is that the opposite of oppression is not a wilderness of litigation and reparation but the nurture of concrete, shared respect."[101]

The more that we, as faith-based individuals, understand about economic, social, and cultural rights, the more effectively we may be able to engage in meaningful conversation toward integrated multidisciplinary efforts for global health, including the nurture of respect. This is true, I believe, even if we ourselves do not always agree on various aspects of the rights-based paradigm. The next two chapters explore complementary approaches that are sometimes more common and commonly supported by faith-based initiatives centering on religious identity. And yet each of these two, also, invites a deeper engagement in the use of human rights for realizing social justice.

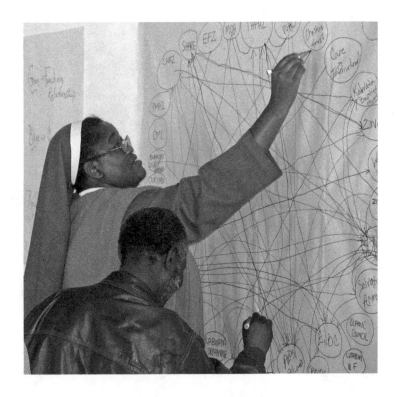

BETWEEN CAPE TOWN

AND MEMPHIS

Religious Health Assets

ONE HOT SUMMER day, three religion professors sat talking in a tin boat on a river near Cape Town, South Africa. It was late December 2002. In the years since apartheid had ended in 1994, the HIV/AIDS epidemic had ravaged Sub-Saharan Africa, destroying communities and undermining many South Africans' hopes for the nation's new freedoms. The three men in the boat— two Congregational ministers who grew up in South Africa and one Anglican priest from Lesotho—had a long collective history as political activists opposed to the oppressions and resulting legacies of the apartheid regime. All three men were white. Their talk that day circled round a recently established faith-based collaborative to connect religion with health care: an initiative called the African Religious Health Assets Programme (ARHAP). The story of ARHAP—its founding vision, research, and influence—is the focus of this chapter. As an example of an international collaborative that is particularly well-documented in the public and online record for its focus on faith-based engagement in poverty, social justice, and health care delivery in settings of poverty, the ARHAP story offers a lens for viewing both the potential and limiting challenges and opportunities of an asset-based approach in global health.[1]

Religion matters deeply in traditional cultures across most of the fifty-four distinct nations in the continent of Africa, and this is also true in the country of South Africa. Faith and spirituality are woven into the moral ideal sometimes expressed as *Ubuntu*—a philosophy of "human kindness" that is occasionally articulated as, "I am what I am because of who we all are."[2] Ubuntu views human community in an intersubjective interconnectedness unlike that of European or Western ideas that distinguish the individual from her or his group or community. Missionary health providers in South Africa have, for example, been part of the public health system since the 1970s. This integral recognition of religion in health did not change when apartheid gave way to democracy in 1994, and the government of South Africa, including its Ministry of Health, continues to recognize the faith-based sector as an integral part of public responses to health issues such as HIV/AIDS. In 2013, for example, the minister of social development stated that:

> all sectors of our society, including FBOs [faith-based organizations] must be mobilised in its entirety to work together to build a caring and proud society, based on shared values and a vision informed by the principles of Ubuntu, human rights and equality, social solidarity, and civic responsibility.[3]

Within this national connectedness, specific religious expression is very diverse. Modern Christianity came to South Africa with colonialism and missionary movements, usually dated around the sixteenth century, and many black South Africans today recognize the troubled heritage that connects the Christian faith with a legacy of subordination and oppression. This legacy has not been helped by "Christian" messages in the 1990s that blamed and stigmatized those across the African continent who were affected by the HIV/AIDS epidemic. While a detailed study of religion and social action under apartheid and in the transition to the post-apartheid era is far beyond the limits of this book, these dynamics of culture and religion are important to keep in mind here as part of the background that shaped—and continues to shape—the ARHAP research collaborative and its influence on faith-based dialogue in public health and health-care delivery across Southern Africa.[4]

ARHAP: A BRIEF HISTORY

The relationships that led to the ARHAP consortium began long before 2002, during the oppressive era of apartheid in South Africa. The oldest of the three men in the boat, James Cochrane, professor of religion at the University of Cape Town (UCT), had converted to Christianity as a teenager in the 1960s, inspired by the legendary Reverend Theo Kotze, who is sometimes called a "liberation theologian."[5] Kotze was a white Methodist minister and anti-apartheid activist who served between 1965 and 1966 as chaplain appointed to political prisoner Robert Sobukwe, the black founder of the Pan-Africanist Congress (PAC) who was then imprisoned (like Nelson Mandela) on Robben Island. Kotze was to remain close to Sobukwe even after Sobukwe was released from prison only to be "banned" (put under house arrest) up until his death on February 27, 1978.[6] In 1968 Kotze co-directed, with Beyers Naudé, the Cape Town office of the Christian Institute (CI); there, Jim Cochrane would later work with Kotze on interracial and justice activities that were often illegal. Naudé, who had founded the CI in South Africa in 1963, was an Afrikaner minister of the conservative Dutch Reformed Church who had repudiated his political and religious ties with the National Party, openly preaching against apartheid after the shock of the 1960 Sharpeville massacre convinced him that he needed to take a public stand whatever the personal cost.[7] Nelson Mandela would later praise Naudé's life as "a shining beacon . . . demonstrat[ing] what it means to rise above race, to be a true South African."[8]

Cochrane would later describe the CI as a community center committed to nonviolent opposition to apartheid. It did this by sharing information, welcoming blacks and whites together in (illegal) shared meals, shared community life, work, and occasional housing. Kotze's vision for the Cape Town office was, Cochrane recalled, that of

> A Church without walls—a church open to all, freely welcoming, without constraints of ideology, dogma or even belief as a condition of that welcome . . . ecumenism based on the unity of praxis, out of credibility of the gospel defended, precisely through a fully inclusive compassion and sense of human dignity that was willing to acknowledge the convictions and gifts of others.[9]

Many in the CI paid dearly for their political and religious opposition to apartheid. Yet, even after the CI was banned in 1977 and Kotze, hidden in the trunk of a car, went into exile, "the inner circle continued to meet illegally . . . in strange places at odd hours."[10]

During the 1980s Cochrane, who would eventually complete theological studies in the United States, and his wife Renate, a Moravian Lutheran pastor and student of theologian Jürgen Moltmann, were active in pushing across racial boundaries and building international networks in South Africa to support faith-based responses to health and justice inequities through their involvement in activist organizations; these included the Institute for Contextual Theology and their support for the United Democratic Front.[11] In 1987, Cochrane helped to establish the School of Theology at the University of Natal, and took a teaching appointment in religious studies at the University of Cape Town. Shortly before ARHAP took shape, one of Cochrane's colleagues and former senior pastor, the Rev. John de Gruchy—a Barth scholar who had also completed doctoral work in the United States on German resistance theologian Dietrich Bonhoeffer—described Cochrane as one who has "long since cast off the piety

of evangelical adolescence and more recently the spiritual barren-
ness of so much political activism."[12]

The other two men in the boat were a generation younger
than Cochrane. Steve de Gruchy (John's son) had been in the
youth group Cochrane launched for teens during his year at
the Rondebosch Congregational (later United) Church in the
Western Cape. Growing up in South Africa, Steve's vision for
the church was profoundly shaped by his father's work, including close ties with the South African Council of Churches. Steve
completed his doctoral research in the late 1980s, on theologian
Reinhold Niebuhr; in 1992 Steve would argue that Niebuhr's
views on race and justice could be "a valuable dialogue partner
in the coming years" for South Africa's emergence from apartheid.[13] As a "religious objector" to compulsory military service
with the South African Defense Force (SADF), Steve had worked
during the late 1980s as a hospital chaplain, observing firsthand
the intersection of religion and health care in South Africa during apartheid.[14] From 1994 to 2000, Steve and his wife, Marian
Loveday, a health-care specialist, directed the Moffat Mission
Trust in Kuruman, Northern Cape,[15] where he "saw what suffering forced removals and the Bantustan policy inflicted on its
victims"[16] and became fluent in Tswana, the local language.[17] In
2000 Steve was named director of the Theology and Development
Programme at the School of Theology at the University of Natal
(now the University of KwaZulu-Natal); he would later head this
university's School of Religion and Theology.[18]

The third man in the boat on that day when Jim Cochrane
invited his young friends to join ARHAP was Paul Germond,
an Anglican priest and one of Steve de Gruchy's oldest friends.
Germond's ancestors had immigrated to Lesotho from
Switzerland as missionaries and teachers in the nineteenth
century.[19] Like Cochrane and the de Gruchys, Germond too spent
time in the United States, briefly studying at Columbia, before
returning to South Africa to teach sociology at the University of
Witwatersrand.

FROM ABCD TO ARHAP

In his teaching at the University of Natal, Steve de Gruchy had been experimenting with what was at that time a new idea in sociology, the "asset-based approach to community development" (ABCD). First described as a distinct method in 1993 by John P. Kretzman and John L. McKnight at the Institute for Policy Research at Northwestern University in Chicago, the ABCD approach was based on community-generated "mapping" of non-fiscal assets (gifts, skills, and capacities) by persons living in poverty in devastated or economically depressed neighborhoods. Kretzman and McKnight's original focus was on low-income communities in the United States. The goal of ABCD was "to help communities not only to recognize and map their assets—the individuals, local associations and institutions which make up the sinew of the neighborhood—but to mobilize them for development purposes."[20] Asset-based community development acknowledges and embraces the strong neighborhood-rooted traditions of community organizing, economic development, and neighborhood planning. Kretzman and McKnight also emphasized that "focusing on the assets of lower income communities does not imply that these communities do not need additional resources from the outside . . . [but rather] that outside resources will be much more effectively used if the local community is itself fully mobilized and invested, and if it can define the agendas for which additional resources must be obtained."

Even though it was not developed for religious purposes, the ABCD model quickly began to influence faith-based groups who were looking for new ideas to affirm respect and dignity in development and mission work with low-income communities both in the United States and abroad.[21] In South Africa, Steve de Gruchy had been impressed by the way this model sparked conversation in the classroom and how it got his theology students thinking about the role of justice in Christian pastoral activities in South Africa.[22]

Indeed, for de Gruchy, a committed scholar and environmentalist, faith issues were inseparable from practical social justice. Later teased by his friends for being "the first person to use the word 'shit' in an academic paper,"[23] Steve would develop these ideas further in his essay on "Water and Spirituality: Theology in a Time of Cholera," delivered at Stellenbosch University on June 25, 2009, reflecting on a cholera epidemic that had killed more than four thousand people in Zimbabwe in 2008 and 2009.[24] Emphasizing the value of religion and public health collaborations, the essay draws on the story of Dr. John Snow and a little-known neighborhood Anglican curate, the Rev. Henry Whitehead, who worked together to solve the 1854 London cholera epidemic. Snow's decision to remove the handle of the Broad Street Pump (where the neighborhood was getting its cholera-infected water) is often seen as the beginning of modern public health.[25] Arguing for the importance of an integrated, consistent, and serious theological framework that can shape responsible environmental ethics today, Steve wrote,

> [T]he truth of the hydrological cycle is that 'we all live down-stream.' There is only one stream of water. What passes through the bodies of humans passes through the bodies of animals, insects and plants. It flushes through our sanitation systems, flows through the rivers, seeps through wetlands, rises to the heavens to become clouds, and returns to nourish us and all living things. There is no life outside this cycle, and theology has to get real about it.[26]

It was the spirit of friendship and a commitment to integrate religion and health in practical action that was to shape and characterize the ARHAP consortium.

ARHAP was formally launched at the Carter Center in Atlanta, Georgia, in April 2002. Ensuing discussions then led to its official "birth" in December that year, in Geneva, Switzerland,[27] between "concerned principles from three continents, assisted by the Health Desk of the World Council of Churches."[28] Its purpose was to

> develop a systematic knowledge base of religious health assets in sub-Saharan Africa to align and enhance the work of religious health leaders and public policy decision-makers in their collaborative effort to meet the challenges of disease, e.g. HIV/AIDS, and to participate in the creation of health, especially for those in poverty.[29]

Most important, the initiative was *not* conceived as "only for Africa." Cochrane has emphasized that ARHAP's intended scope was "quite distinctly a global one, with international partners (who had met in Geneva), but beginning in Africa, on the grounds of a determination to reverse the usual flow of knowledge and sources of investigation." That is, instead of exogenous input—the usual direction of missions and aid *to* Africa from somewhere else—in ARHAP an African initiative would reach out, with its global partners *from Africa* to the world. The later name change from ARHAP to IRHAP (International Religious Health Assets Programme) was intended to further this vision in a deliberate attempt "both to reflect its actual work, and to overcome the 'prejudice' among many that ARHAP was 'only for Africa.'"[30] While clearly based in South Africa, the focus of work insofar as it did relate to the continent looked outward across all of Sub-Saharan Africa.

The founding members—principal investigators on the initial research proposal—included Cochrane and two Americans at Emory: Gary R. Gunderson and Deborah McFarland. McFarland was a Peace Corps veteran and public health researcher at Emory's Rollins School of Public Health, who had previously worked for the Centers for Disease Control (CDC) in Atlanta and who remains active in faith-based health dialogue at Emory to the present. Gunderson, an ordained Baptist minister with particular gifts in health-care administration, had directed the Interfaith Health Program (IHP), an initiative launched in 1992 at the Carter Center "to assist faith groups in reaching disadvantaged populations with health care information."[31] IHP—which moved to Emory in 1999—had been founded by Bill Foege, a medical doctor also trained in public health. The son of a Lutheran minister, Foege became famous while he was a medical missionary for his work on the global campaign to eradicate smallpox in West and Central Africa.[32] As Foege's successor at IHP, Gunderson also worked closely with faith-based organizations and health programs in several African countries, including participation in events that Cochrane had organized over the years at the University of Cape Town.[33] Gunderson knew Kretzman and McKnight and their ABCD work, and it was Gunderson who, at ARHAP's 2002 launch, proposed the need for research on "religious health assets" that was to become the signature of ARHAP's fieldwork and focus.

From the start the group was starkly honest about the concern that religion could also be a problem in health-care-related action. In drafting ARHAP's "Framing Document," they addressed this concern by noting that "a naïve view of the role of religion would undermine our grasp of the necessary social realities; hence we recognize the need to balance the positive with a clear grasp of the limits and possible negative impact of religious traditions or faith-based practices in particular contexts."[34]

The collaborative would maintain its commitment to begin in Africa and reach outward. By the time of Steve de Gruchy's tragic death, in February 2010, ARHAP research teams in South Africa were based at three Collaborative Centres. Jim Cochrane was director at the hub, at the University of Cape Town, de Gruchy at the School of Religion and Theology at the University of KwaZulu-Natal, and Paul Germond at Witwatersrand University, in collaboration with Dr. Liz Thomas, a research expert on social capital and the health of women, who was based at the Centre for Health Policy. Across the Atlantic, Gunderson and McFarland launched a similar team of colleagues, with the focus moving with Gunderson, first to Memphis, Tennessee, where he directed Methodist LeBonheur Healthcare, and in 2012 to Wake Forest, North Carolina, with his appointment as vice president of faith and health ministries. ARHAP also established an independent board of directors that included globally respected figures such as the South African feminist theologian, Denise Ackermann, and Francis Wilson, a leading lay Anglican and economist on issues of migrant labor, poverty, and inequality.

The Geneva-based World Health Organization (WHO) soon became a third player in ARHAP's vision and action, through Gunderson's acquaintance with an Episcopal priest, the Rev. Canon Ted Karpf.[35] A longtime HIV/AIDS activist and canon at the Washington (DC) National Cathedral, Karpf had worked with the World Council of Churches in Geneva in the 1970s, then with the Anglican archbishop in South Africa since 2000, visiting hundreds of parishioners across twenty-three dioceses as part of an effort toward strategic planning to address the HIV/AIDS challenge.[36] In 2004, he moved back to Geneva, invited by Dr. Jim Yong Kim, who was then advisor to World Health Organization Director General Lee Jong Wook. Kim (later appointed president of the World Bank) was then directing the "3 by 5" initiative, launched by WHO together with the Joint United Nations Programme on HIV/AIDS (UNAIDS), with an aim to reach three million HIV-positive persons in low- and middle-income countries with effective antiretroviral (ARV) treatment by 2005.[37]

RESEARCH-BASED ACTION

ARHAP's consortium of health and religion professionals, activists, practitioners, and graduate students, gradually began to develop through the production of research and writing that was driven by a shared passion for faith-based social justice and community health. In practice the collaboration was not particularly hierarchical despite its named "leaders." Working within a central operational structure at the University of Cape Town, with general direction and research administration by a faculty team consisting of Cochrane together with Barbara Schmid and Jill Olivier, and managed by a group ranging from sixteen to twenty faculty, students, and practitioners, ARHAP's researchers and invited colleagues and guest speakers from Africa, North America, and Europe met as often as they could on a shoestring budget to share and develop ideas and to explore ways to translate their work into real-life practice that would make a difference for affected communities. The Americans in the group participated in the meetings in South Africa and worked to apply ARHAP principles to health-related issues in low-income neighborhoods back in the United States. Both regional contingents welcomed and shared graduate students who were interested in working on the different sites.

As WHO Partnerships Officer, Ted Karpf was excited about the collaborative. He was especially excited by ARHAP's commitment to produce "evidence-based" research, something that was also a WHO priority. As a clergyman in health activism, he was also excited that the consortium sought to document the effects of religious values on practical health-related activities. In 2005 several ARHAP researchers were completing what would become ARHAP's first project, a systematic review and research report on the "Masangane" AIDS treatment program in a remote, arid, and impoverished region in the Eastern Cape. This study, funded by the Vesper Society, was especially important to ARHAP's focus on evidence because it looked at the role of systematic monitoring and evaluation to measure whether an intervention actually does what it promises. Such evaluation studies are often missing in health-funded research, especially faith-based projects. Direct care organizations often feel more obligated to use their limited budgets to deliver services rather than take time and pay staff for follow-up evaluation based on (what is often hurried and partial) recordkeeping. Yet evaluation is crucial in research. It helps document whether resources were used responsibly, preventing tragic waste of time, efforts, and ultimately human lives if something does not "work." For programs that seem to be effective (at least for the few people they serve), evaluations can help shape and justify decisions about what to do better. ARHAP's commitment to an evaluation and review of the Masangane program set an important precedent.

Masangane (meaning "let us embrace") began in 1996, when a South African Moravian nurse, Sister Jabu Sikhonje, realized that she was seeing an increasing number of young women who were diagnosed with both tuberculosis and HIV/AIDS.[38] In response to this growing crisis, Mama Magoloza, a Sunday School teacher in the region, was trained to provide HIV/AIDS education and awareness through church groups, Bible studies, medical support (including condoms), and community care to serve the sick, the discouraged, and the dying. South African and Xhosa-speaking pastors made up the program's initial leaders, including Ntombentsha Matinisi, the first Xhosa woman pastor in the Moravian church in South Africa. With help from the Rev. Renate Cochrane, the group was able to get outside funding and administrative support. By 2001 Masangane was paying for school fees and uniforms for HIV/AIDS orphans. The program was intentionally kept small since resources were very limited and the region extremely remote; it could not afford to advertise or attract more people than it could help. From 1996 to 2002, the program had no medications available to treat HIV/AIDS, and it consisted entirely of education, efforts at prevention, palliative treatment, and care for surviving children. The resource potential for treatment changed in 2003, with South Africa's national "roll-out" plan for distributing antiretroviral medications.

Yet effective drug therapy for HIV/AIDS is a lifelong need. If a person cannot get the drugs they require each day, their health will suffer. Inconsistent treatment may foster drug resistance. And if someone who catches a drug-resistant form of the disease infects others, entire communities could soon be facing an epidemic disaster. This is why keeping the Masangane treatment program small seemed the best option for helping the community. In 2002 a retired school principal, the Rev. Fikile Mgcoyi, took leadership of the Masangane program, maintaining tight fiscal control until his death in 2005. As soon as ARVs were available, Masangane's personalized attention to its cohort and its faith-based connections made it possible to ensure that its HIV-positive participants got onto ARV therapy much faster than they would have in the government's program. Medical coverage was an ongoing challenge; as late as 2005, ARV was *available* (in theory) in only 62 percent of the country's public health facilities; in fact, less than 20 percent of those in need actually received treatment.[39] But Masangane participants could get treatment as soon as they were enrolled. Masangane also ensured that drug adherence was high, thanks to home visits, a buddy system, and weekly support groups. While most clients were not members of a particular church, the communities as a whole were deeply religious, and most identified with the Christian faith. Regardless of religious practices, participants welcomed the program's spiritual support, which included the practice of timing daily spiritual reading and prayer as a reminder for taking one's medication.[40]

The ARHAP evaluation—of whether and how well Masangane was actually working—coincided with a leadership crisis that erupted after Mgcoyi's death. Many of the most effective workers had found jobs elsewhere, and recordkeeping and accounting for funds had become more relaxed. As usually happens in low-budget faith-based programs, only a few people on the Masangane staff were paid, and most of the work was done by volunteers. The volunteers were former program participants, people living with HIV/AIDS (PLWAs), who received a small travel allowance and did the work because of their personal commitments to helping others in the community.

The paradox of expecting people who are extremely poor to work for free in community health is a common practice in many non-sectarian and faith-based NGOs. However, there are strong reasons to argue that such community health workers not only deserve to be paid but should and must be paid.[41] ARHAP's evaluation report identified this as a serious problem, noting that, "It has been Masangane's experience that one cannot sustainably use volunteers who are unemployed and have no income."[42] The program was later able to purchase two vehicles to help make travel easier, but did not significantly alter the volunteer reimbursement. The ARHAP reviewers advised that "urgent consideration needs to be given to the financial arrangement needed to provide sustainable ARV treatment to the current and future Masangane beneficiaries."[43]

The report was a sobering, instructive, and frank look at a struggling community-based effort that was seriously challenged by forced transition. The program would indeed survive (it is still loosely affiliated with the Moravian church[44]), but following Rev. Mgcoyi's death, its funding and personalized investment in community accompaniment would not be the same. For ARHAP, the report was also an apt transition, marking it as a committed group moving beyond its early enthusiasm into a new era of active research and funding.

Ted Karpf worked to help ARHAP apply for a WHO grant that would underwrite its next research project: to test an asset-based participatory research model that Steve de Gruchy and the ARHAP team had created and playfully dubbed PIRHANA: Participatory Inquiry into Religious Health Assets, Networks and Agency. Piloted by de Gruchy, his doctoral student Sinatra Matimelo, and other ARHAP researchers in Zambia in 2005, the PIRHANA toolset consisted of intensive participatory workshops in which both "health providers" and "health seekers" asked questions, created literal maps and connecting diagrams (see the image that opens this chapter) of local community-based asset-related resources, and analyzed the results with a focus on evidence for what the communities identified as effective connections between religion and health.

WHO funding allowed ARHAP to perform a detailed research project in two countries, Zambia and Lesotho. The resulting report, *Appreciating Assets: The Contribution of Religion to Universal Access in Africa* (Cape Town, 2006), was officially released at a public relations event in the National Cathedral in Washington, DC, in February 2007, under the auspices of the WHO and chaired by its then executive director.[45] "To anyone's knowledge," Cochrane recalls, "it was (and probably remains) the first time the WHO, strongly averse like all UN organizations to any 'religious complicity,' held such a gathering in a religious building."[46] Before long, other research groups also began to use the PIRHANA toolset for similar research.[47]

ASSETS AND THE "HEALTHWORLD"

Both the Masangane and 2006 PIRHANA study embodied two essential concepts that express ARHAP's very particular approach to the integration of religion with health. The first, based on McKnight and Kretzman's model but tweaked substantially, is that of *religious health assets*. The second is the idea of the *healthworld*, a phrase that Cochrane and Germond developed to "translate" for their American and European readers certain concepts inherent in traditional African community health that are important for other cultures as well.

Religious Health Assets

The idea of religious health assets began by looking at intangible or non-economic assets: that is, ways those in poor communities help one another. Such transactional behaviors outside the fiscal marketplace can include, for example, donations, subsidies, fee-for-service, loans, sharing, redistribution, cooperation, and intervention (prayer and conflict resolution are two examples of intervention). While material help might include money, goods, or productive assets (like tools and seeds), non-material help can take the form of knowledge (advice, information, transfer of skills), physical or manual support (shelter, transport, protection), moral/emotional support (prayer, comfort, encouragement, and solidarity), or intervention (to help address problems, decisions, and conflicts).[48]

ARHAP's PIRHANA toolset drew on this basic understanding of assets and expanded it to include community resources where religion and health intersect, illustrated in Table 5.1.

In the field, they asked workshop participants to tell them, "What does religion contribute to health?" Answers varied, and included: hope, faith, prayer, temperance, compassion, healing/health services, material support for orphans and vulnerable children, and advocacy. The 2006 report grouped these answers into seven broad clusters: spiritual encouragement, compassionate care, moral formation, curative intervention, knowledge giving, material support, and public engagement (see Table 5.2).

It is important for religious health and health policy experts to understand why assets matter, said de Gruchy in 2006, because:

> outsiders have pushed deficit thinking and deficit policies onto Africa, and many inside and outside Africa have come to internalise this. Yet graduate students from Africa know and feel a different reality. They know that there are so many assets in Africa and that Africa's future lies in tapping into, protecting, and enhancing these assets—as the basis for global engagement.[49]

Denise M. Ackermann would later emphasize the importance of both critical wisdom and creative risk in how one "does" justice. "When justice is sought in a particular place and for particular reasons," she said, "understanding the context is pivotal for actions that can make a difference. . . . To hope is to live with

Table 5.1

ARHAP THEORY MATRIX: RELIGIOUS HEALTH ASSETS

	Direct Health Outcomes	Indirect Health Outcomes
Intangible	Prayer	Individual
	Resilience	(sense of meaning)
	Health-seeking behavior	Belonging—human/divine
	Motivation	Access to power/energy
	Responsibility	Trust/distrust
	Commitment/sense of duty	Faith-hope-love
	Relationship: caregiver & "patient"	Sacred space in a polluting world
	Advocacy/prophetic	Time
	Resistance: Physical and/ or structural/ political	Emplotment (story)
Tangible	Infrastructure	Manyano & other fellowships
	Hospitals, beds, etc.	Choir
	Clinics	Education
	Dispensaries	Sacraments/rituals
	Training-paramedical	Rites of passage
	Hospices	(accompanying)
	Funding/development agencies	Funerals
	Holistic support	Network/connections
	Hospital chaplains	Leadership skills
	Faith healers	Presence in the "Bundu"
	Traditional healers	(on the margins)
	Care groups	Boundaries (Normative)
	NGO/FBO—"projects"	

Source: James R. Cochrane and Barbara Schmid eds., *ARHAP Tools Workshop Report* (Cape Town: June 6–8, 2004), 6. Reprinted with permission.

Table 5.2

RELIGIOUS HEALTH ASSETS: "WHAT DOES RELIGION CONTRIBUTE TO HEALTH?"

Respondents' terms	ARHAP conceptual "cluster"
Hope, faith, spiritual counseling/ support, prayer, trust, baptism, salvation, peace	Spiritual encouragement
Care and support/compassion, love, well-being, holistic health	Compassionate care
Behavior change, life/positive living, patience, temperance, moral guidance, self-control, morality	Moral formation
Unity, respect, belonging	Respectful relationships
Healing/health services, infrastructure, human resources	Curative intervention
Sensitization/teaching, education, instruction, awareness	Knowledge giving
Material support/orphan and vulnerable children (OVC) support, food	Material support
Advocacy	Public engagement

Adapted from African Religious Health Assets Programme (ARHAP) under contract to the World Health Organization. *Appreciating Assets: The Contribution of Religion to Universal Access in Africa; Mapping, Understanding, Translating, and Engaging Religious Health Assets in Zambia and Lesotho in Support of Universal Access to HIV/AIDS Treatment, Care and Prevention* (Cape Town: ARHAP, October 2006), drawing on data at pp. 76–77 (for Zambia) and pp. 111–112 (for Lesotho).

expectation, undergirded by patience, in a creative manner that commits us to actions for justice."[50]

The ARHAP model is not about cookie-cutter solutions. Gunderson emphasized that religious health assets

> are fragile and unstable and personal. But they emerge and thrive in most amazing way[s]. The more we understand this vital logic, the less we will fear the apparent fragility. . . . The more we pay attention to connection and allow our own complex connections to work, the more we will understand about these living assets and the more alive we will be.[51]

Healthworld

When the third man in the tin boat, Paul Germond, set out with his student researchers to map assets in Lesotho, the team began by asking people in the local communities how they understood religion and health. At the end of the first day, they realized that the question made no sense in the local language because no word existed to differentiate religion from health. However, there was one word—*bophelo*—that people in Lesotho seemed to use in a way that encompassed both ideas. Roughly translated as communal well-being, bophelo in fact contains deep nuances that encompass a broad range of everything that makes one well. Health is grounded in a relational dynamic to the entire community, including rituals, ancestors, and even the function of local architecture. The village post office, for example, people told them, contributes to community and individual bophelo since there one can receive mail that contains money sent from relatives working in the cities, and it also serves as the local bank.[52] A related concept common in South Africa today is that of Ubuntu, discussed above.

This insight led Cochrane and Germond to coin a new English term, *healthworld*, as a cognate for a traditional, indeed age-old idea, but one that is often unknown or poorly understood in Europe, North America, and much of modern Western culture. One's healthworld is the manner in which one understands the relationship between health, wellness, faith, and deity in a particular conceptual network of interrelated ideas and assumptions. The ARHAP concept of healthworld may be contrasted with the common views about health in the modern West. A medical missionary from the Global North and an atheist physicist trained, say, in New Zealand, might, for example, share a common perspective about their health based in assumptions about the separation of matter from "spirit" such that (even if the atheist disbelieves in "spirit") they would understand one another perfectly. However, this separation might make no sense to a rural fisherman, cattle farmer, or traditional healer or mine worker in Sub-Saharan Africa or Southeast Asia, for whom the universe, body, spirit, and ancestors all flow together in quite a different conceptual manner. In Europe and the West, for example, an individual is believed capable of being "in perfect health" even when her or his family, work, and social environment are deeply dysfunctional and even pathological. But in Lesotho (as in many other cultures), individual "health" is so bound up with the whole community, past and present, that "perfect health" requires action at both individual and community levels, perhaps including prescriptive rituals. An HIV-positive person who cannot access antiretroviral therapy might claim "perfect health" if the local healers and community consider him or her to be in proper social harmony regardless of how a laboratory blood test might measure viral status. These different ways to see health inevitably shape responses to health-care delivery in different cultures. The idea of the healthworld forces recognition of these differences even as it advances the idea that all factors (physical, spiritual, social, environmental) must be considered together as a single concept impacting one's health. Healthworld, in other words, "encompasses a consideration of physical, mental and spiritual health, across both individuals and groups (the family, the nation), rather than just the absence of disease at individual level."[53] ARHAP's Masangane study, for example, emphasized that healthworld

> [i]ncorporates peoples' conceptions of health, their health seeking behaviour, and the conditions of health that affect them. These conditions are shaped by health policies of governments, the variety of health practices within a given region, the interaction between health and religious practices, and the social and environmental determinants of health.[54]

Gunderson deliberately applied the healthworld concept to his work at Wake Forest in the United States. He named the new division's magazine *FaithHealth*, explaining in his first editorial that this deliberately unified word was meant to dissolve "the distinction between spiritual care, medical care, community health, counseling and the health of congregations."[55]

TRANSITION AND TRAGEDY

Between 2006 and 2011, ARHAP's research output was impressive. In 2006 Dr. Jill Olivier and her Cape Town colleagues, with editorial support from the Emory team faculty, published a near-encyclopedic literature review and bibliography.[56] ARHAP funding from Tearfund and UNAIDS supported a report in 2009, *The potential and perils of partnership: Christian religious entities and collaborative stakeholders responding to HIV in Kenya, Malawi and the DRC.* That report identified gaps and highlighted the ongoing potential for advancing a UNAIDS policy of "Three Ones." This is a policy intended to make all interventions as consistent and useful as possible, with: (1) interventions coordinated under a single action framework, (2) a single national coordinating authority, and (3) a single monitoring and evaluation system.[57]

A grant from the Bill & Melinda Gates Foundation supported a "landscaping study," a more detailed description of faith-based organizations in Sub-Saharan Africa, published in 2008.[58] Based on extensive interviews, focus groups, and case studies from Zambia, Uganda, and Mali, the Gates report identified key areas for investment and "scale-up" (revising and expanding apparently successful programs to serve more people). For the Gates research, as for the earlier research, ARHAP's team members focused on listening in order to represent voices and needs most accurately. As Gunderson put it in 2005, "Listening; in a way that's all ARHAP is—a listening project straining to hear the birdsong amid the jets, the heartbeat of life amid the cries of cruel and vastly premature death."[59]

The Gates report described a historical moment ripe with opportunities for change.[60] Religion could be an asset for community health across Africa, the report concluded—and one with immense potential for improvement. Religious leaders were an important underutilized resource for health promotion that was often channeled into some creative but poorly supported initiatives.

The Gates study was also important for attracting global attention from health policy and funding experts. Having such an international high-profile funding source, ARHAP's researchers affirmed for the public the value of taking an interest in religion in Sub-Saharan Africa. As a result, the report could be a useful lobbying tool to help establish increased resource support and collaboration for effective health-care delivery.

The report's timing, however, was unfortunate. Published just as the global economic market took a nosedive, the report left ARHAP faced with what must have felt like an abrupt black hole, just as the work seemed to be finding its global voice, and training a diaspora of graduate students as well as new clergy and faculty across several continents. In February 2010 the group suffered a more personal loss, when Steve de Gruchy died suddenly in a whitewater rafting accident, devastating his friends, family, and colleagues. Given these economic and team-based transitions,

ARHAP faced significant challenges to moving forward in the context of the tragedy of loss that included a new global economic climate.

Subtle shifts followed over the next few years. James Cochrane officially retired, but continued as nominal director across team collaborations, in addition to working with Gunderson on "Leading Causes of Life" (discussed further below) as well as helping to generate a prolific flow of publications.[61] In part to signal this transitional phase while affirming ongoing continuity, the collaborative entered a new partnership, in 2011. Renamed IRHAP, it became a component of the University of Cape Town's School of Public Health and Family Medicine. Dr. Jill Olivier—who had been a core team participant in ARHAP research from the start—took the helm as director of research and publications, working closely together with IRHAP co-directors, Cochrane and Professor Lucy Gilson.

ASSETS AND GLOBAL HEALTH IN THE AMERICAN BIBLE BELT

Meanwhile, in the United States, ARHAP's two other co-founders, Gary Gunderson and Deborah McFarland at Emory, continued to foster collaborative research in the context of the American health-care system. Indeed, the Interfaith Health Program at Emory reflected another type of local community. IHP had been founded during what some called the "Welfare Revolution" in America, during the years between President Bill Clinton's 1996 welfare reform legislation—which undercut a broad range of social services that had been available to the unemployed—and President George W. Bush's Charitable Choice Act of 2001, a deliberate appeal to faith-based organizations to help fill the gaps in social services at both local and national levels (often by eliminating government funds while appealing to a volunteer ethic). As noted above, such a focus on volunteerism is a controversial practice that the Masangane reviewers as well as many others insist is unsustainable in settings of poverty.[62]

Under Gunderson's leadership, the American-based research would likewise focus on mobilizing religious groups as health-care networks linking low-income, high-risk hospitalized patients with the resources they need to reenter the community, live healthy lives, and avoid rapid readmission rates back into the hospital. In 2007 ARHAP partnered with Emory's Religion and Public Health Collaborative (RPHC) to map and mobilize religious health assets in refugee and immigrant communities in two metro Atlanta neighborhoods. Sinatra Matimelo, a former banker and Baptist pastor from Zambia who had worked closely with de Gruchy as a graduate student on the original research, spent time with the Emory group to help develop a version of the PIRHANA tool that would be culturally appropriate in a US-based setting.[63]

Meanwhile, Gunderson was appointed senior vice president of Methodist LeBonheur Healthcare in Memphis, Tennessee, where he would continue his faculty affiliation with Emory until his appointment at Wake Forest in 2011. While advancing the vision for religious health assets, Gunderson's research focused more on "boundary leadership" and what he would come to call the "leading causes of life." This phrase was intended to counter the more common tendency in medicine and public health epidemiology to focus on pathology or "leading causes of illness" or "death."[64] "Faith is more like health than it is like disease," he argued, "so it requires different questions."

Gunderson approached these questions by suggesting that those who shape health policy begin by listening to how patients themselves view life. First, he suggested, ask a patient to identify the leading causes of their life—what helps them thrive with vitality? Their answer will suggest the things that are really important in working "toward a pattern of connection, coherence, agency, blessing, and hope."[65] Second, health policy makers can gain from asking, "In what ways are religious-social networks and structures assets for health?" Policies and practices developed out of the answers to these two questions, he argued, can shape "a language of life that illustrates what the doctor is working *with*, not just *against*."[66]

Gunderson's approach had more in common with a community health worker (CHW) model that one usually sees in low-income countries rather than across the United States. In the United States, CHWs face severe funding challenges, even when it can be proved that they save money for the health care system and that they can significantly improve health outcomes. In Southern Africa, ARHAP researchers had always been attentive to community structure and "outpatient" health workers such as nurses, CHWs, and peer volunteers. This was partly because there were so few doctors, especially for the poor and black communities, and also because of the colonialist or missionary-based tendency to pay local workers little or nothing. The HIV/AIDS epidemic— affecting largely (but not exclusively) the black population—converged in South Africa with severe historical disparities in health care services.

These disparities remain stark. In the South African context, they had become far worse as a result of the dominant political power dynamics that shaped apartheid policies. According to a study by the late Dr. Phillip V. Tobias, one-time dean of the University of Witwatersrand Medical School and a trenchant critic of apartheid, the number of trained white doctors per million white persons in the South African population in the late 1970s was 142; the number of trained black doctors per million black persons during roughly the same period (1975) was 4.8.[67] During the 1980s, large numbers of trained white South African physicians left South Africa for higher paying jobs in other countries, but the inequities remained. The end of apartheid in 1994 abolished legal segregation, but not the poverty that continued (and continues) to hinder many South African blacks from expecting access to the kind of advanced medical and hospital care that white persons in the United States today often take for granted. As a result, ARHAP research in South Africa had little to do with circumstances related to hospital conditions; it was, instead, usually limited to outpatient clinics and an emphasis on (unpaid) community health workers visiting persons at home.

In the United States, on the other hand, ARHAP principles and research took shape in the direct context of the hospitals and medical centers that represent the dominant American model. As a result, Gunderson's focus on applying ARHAP principles in Atlanta and Memphis from the start concerned conditions related to hospital admissions and discharge. "What do hospitals have to do with health?" he asked at the 2007 ARHAP Colloquium meeting in Cape Town. He was frank about the complex challenges of affirming religion in a hospital setting: "At every scale of human relationship, religious character may be—it often is—a liability . . . contributing to active and passive complicity that obstructs optimal health. Religion can also be—it often is—an asset that helps the internal function of an institution."[68]

In Memphis, Gunderson began to apply these ideas to practical clinical medicine. Methodist LeBonheur Healthcare provided a high percentage of care to the poor throughout Tennessee, and religion is an important aspect of life for many who live in poor communities in America's southeastern Bible Belt. Poverty, poor health, and race are deeply interconnected in the United States, and black Americans face marked disparities in hospital health-care services compared to white Americans.[69] Black Southerners also retain a certain warranted suspicion of the health-care system, remembering ethical abuses such as the infamous Tuskegee "experiment," which allowed thousands of black American men to die of untreated syphilis as late as 1972.[70] These suspicions meant that most of the patients with the greatest medical and economic needs, Gunderson knew, came to the hospital for care late, often with very advanced, late-stage health conditions and risks. However, they were usually persons who identified with a religious tradition or practice, most commonly a Christian church. Building on these affiliations and identities was an opportunity to create innovative liaisons. With help from the medical community, willing congregations and congregants could gain skills to support communications and care related to discharge and staying healthy at home after a hospital admission. The congregational model is also one that tends to function on a largely volunteer ethic. To see what might happen if churches got involved in addressing the health-care gaps related to social determinants of health and illness, Gunderson and his colleagues developed a faith and health community partnership, the Congregational Health Network (CHN).

Under the direction of the Rev. Bobby Baker, a black clergyman from the local community, the Memphis CHN, founded in 2006, facilitated a formal voluntary "covenant" affiliation between the hospital and religious institutions (church, synagogue, mosque, or temple) in the greater Memphis area. Most of the congregations who first joined the network represented urban, low-income African Americans. Once a congregation chose to participate, they would sign a covenant committing to a formal liaison between the hospital and the congregations (which in Memphis are mostly Christian churches). Paid hospital "navigators" under the CHN program director would then develop and work with a network of congregations and their church-member volunteers, called "liaisons." The overwhelming majority of volunteers, Gunderson would later note, are women who also work, full- or part-time, in the health care sector. By 2012 the Memphis CHN served a regional total of more than thirteen thousand congregants.[71] As part of the covenant, the hospital agreed to train each congregation's clergy and the volunteer liaisons. Congregational members who received medical care at the hospital could choose, if they wished, to register their faith affiliation and specific congregation in the hospital electronic medical record (EMR). If they did, a hospital admission would automatically trigger a chain of communications between navigators and liaisons, who would then work together to prepare a personalized support plan for the patient's hospital discharge. Community-based social services depended entirely on individual needs, and might include transportation, meals, shopping, medication pickup, and times when those fellow congregants known to the patient were willing to simply stay with her or him for a few hours when unknown home health providers (e.g., visiting nurses, meal services, grocery deliveries) came knocking.

According to Baker, the CHN program as it continues today commits the hospital to fund training classes for entire congregations. Congregations and their members may enroll in modules that can help them feel comfortable and familiar with the hospital process. Classes include, for example, information on making hospital visits, caring for the dying, mental health "first aid" tips for non-professionals, practical training in how to transfer people from a wheelchair to a car, changing beds, recognizing one's personal limits, and finding out about other community resources available to help. This innovative approach to patient advocacy aims to improve people's journey through the health-care system.[72]

Despite the known tensions over religious volunteerism, the CHN distinction between paid hospital employees and volunteer congregational liaisons is deliberate, said Dr. Teresa Cutts, who worked as director of research for innovation at Methodist LeBonheur before joining Gunderson at the new Wake Forest program in 2013. A hospital that pays community health workers can also lay them off, she argued, but "if someone does something for love and not money, you decrease the incentive if you start to pay them." Supporting this theory, Gunderson noted, "I think it is the liaisons that are moving the data."[73] In other words, the CHN volunteers (who differ from community health workers in many poor countries because they generally also hold down paying jobs) are seen as fostering a sense of community good-neighborliness that is rooted in shared religious identity, a "beholdenness" which evokes identification grounded in concepts of spiritual family.

The Memphis CHN program has demonstrated measurable cost effectiveness. A sample study compared a group of CHN participants with a similar cohort of Memphis-area church members who spent time in the hospital but were not part of the network. The comparison found a significant difference in mortality rates, risk for repeat admissions, and total health-care costs for care. Not only were CHN members half as likely to die during the study period, but they also reported higher levels of patient satisfaction with their medical care. The Memphis program cost $200,000 to develop and $500,000 per year to maintain, the study reported, but it generated an impressive profit of an estimated $4 million.[74] The Memphis program has inspired a number of similar initiatives and inquiries in other cities. At Wake Forest by 2014, Gunderson and Cutts were engaged in replicating the Memphis model, with a vision for a Congregational Health Network touching on several cities and communities across North Carolina. Their work also remains closely linked with the University of Cape Town, as Cochrane, now working from Cape Town and Germany, directs the Leading Causes of Life Initiative, an effort that aims "to develop the basic theory, language and paradigm on which programs can be built to systematically advance life at community scale."[75]

ARHAP's Memphis model also confronts, at least in part, the deeper and more fundamental failure of the American health care system to provide basic social services to those who need support to negotiate the gap between everyday "good" health and the occasional realities of acute in-hospital care. Most Americans today live in this space. These problems and gaps create what public health expert Dr. Elizabeth H. Bradley and her co-author Lauren Taylor have recently called *The American Health Care Paradox*.[76] In most of the world's leading economies, say Bradley and Taylor, every government dollar spent on citizens' health care is paired with two dollars spent on social services; but in the United States the social service expenditure per health-care dollar is a mere sixty cents.[77] This gap affects everyone, not just those who are poor. The life expectancy and health of a country directly correlates with this recipe for government health-care spending, Bradley argues, posing a challenge to think differently about how we do health in the

United States. Effective health insurance not only covers doctors and hospital visits, but also considers the things that make it possible for us to stay healthy after we go home: housing, nutrition, community health-care workers and home-care access, trusted neighbors and friendships, employment, and other related social services. Regardless of whether these needs are filled by paid or volunteer resources, who pays, and how, they are vital, and directly relevant to the social determinants of health and economic, social, and cultural rights discussed in Chapter 4. The Memphis model offers one glimpse at how this gap between a traditionally medical or clinical model of health-care services and what people really need to stay healthy might be addressed in some settings.[78]

THINKING BEYOND ARHAP

At Steve de Gruchy's memorial service in 2010, Jim Cochrane recalled how, "For the last seven years Steve worked closely and pivotally with this highly creative group of friends and colleagues, a task into which I first drew him and Paul one hot December day sitting in a tin boat on a river at Vermaaklikheid, Steve's family holiday home not too far from Cape Town."[79] This chapter has explored the background, context, and ongoing potential of that summertime conversation through the lens of these "three men in the boat" as they engaged in the development of a vibrant multi-player collaborative partnership among researchers, academics, practitioners, and graduate students across several countries, continents, languages, races, and cultures.

The ARHAP story speaks directly to the residual tensions that public health and humanitarian aid experts often feel about the presence of others—coworkers or community members—who make personal statements about religious views and identity. But what are the limits and potential challenges of the ARHAP research itself as it might be applied to other settings? What might we learn from the ARHAP story, whether we affiliate with these ideas as health professionals, as persons of faith who care about justice and health equity, or some combination of these perspectives? How might we read "between" or "under" the narrative history of this particular story to locate points that matter to us but that may not appear evident at first glance?

Thinking beyond the ARHAP story, it seems to me important to keep in mind that ARHAP was only a small piece in global health activities of its own time as well as within its broader historical context. I have focused this chapter on its example as a cameo "case," a story that captures the essence of one set of practices related to "just belief" as they are being lived out among a particular group of real people in real time in the twenty-first century. But the ARHAP model cannot be generalized as the only approach to faith-based responses to poverty, or even the only approach to religious health assets.

The ARHAP collaboration—its coherence and its story—also depended largely on a very particular and perhaps even unique window in international global health funding. It started with a high-profile disease trigger (HIV/AIDS and its global health risks as they were affecting social interactions in Sub-Saharan Africa on a massive population level), a particular stage in HIV/AIDS diagnostic and treatment research, and a particular window of global interest in religion and society followed by September 11, 2001, combined with a particularly optimistic era in multilateral funding organizations for health, an optimism seriously challenged by the worldwide economic crises of late 2009. As a story, the ARHAP narrative is perhaps like all good stories, both unique in its detail and rich in themes that it shares in common with other aspects of what it is to be human. Reduced (or redirected) global funding now poses new questions and challenges. How might ARHAP/IRHAP move forward to advance and also apply this wealth of information in an apparently more grants-scarce environment? How could researchers from other philosophical or religious traditions apply it to other cultures? What would such research and participatory engagement look like, for example, in South America? China? Saudi Arabia? The Middle East?

The ARHAP vision and context is also rooted in a very particular mix of national cultures and histories. Behind ARHAP's founders in South Africa, we can glimpse the influence of colonialism, missionary health-related activities rooted in the nineteenth century, the ecumenical movement as it shaped global religious dialogue and social action in the 1950s and 1960s, racial disparities, tensions, and reactions related to the apartheid regime between the 1970s and 1990s, and a South African diaspora that fostered networking and multicultural experiences among Africa, Europe, and the United States. Both de Gruchy and Cochrane have taken great pains to deliberately identify these risks and tensions, and to emphasize the importance of culturally contextualized agency and participation.[80] But the threads indelibly remain. ARHAP's significance for health policy dialogue today really cannot be separated from at least some consideration of these foundational influences.

ARHAP and its research fits best into health dialogues relevant to cultural settings where religion and religious identity have deep roots and intrinsic and widely recognized social value. Germond and Cochrane's research on healthworld and the idea of bophelo in Lesotho is just one example. Most of the African communities in ARHAP's research self-identify with a religion, in most cases Christianity. Christian faith-based convictions and practices also inform the co-founders' history of their sometimes radical social action (such as illegal activism during apartheid and the ecumenical model of the Christian Institute).

These observations are not intended as criticism, but rather as a caution for those who might rush without thought into building new ideas and practices intended to copy this model. Indeed, ARHAP team members were acutely conscious of this parochial dimension and the questions and challenges it raised for ARHAP's relevance in settings and collegial partnerships that might be marked by greater religious diversity. In 2007, for example, participant reflections suggested that not everyone felt their religious concerns were represented within the overall project. Discussants admitted that "Many who enter public health do so because they were damaged by religion or were driven out by their own tradition," recommending that ARHAP researchers "Keep research basic enough to allow people who have been scarred by religion to hear what you say to be able to intervene in areas of public health."[81] Early on in the research, one participating anthropologist, Fiona Scorgie of the University of KwaZulu-Natal, identified a number of problems she perceived that might handicap ARHAP's relevance for health professionals and others who don't identify with traditional Christianity. A faith-based approach such as ARHAP, Scorgie argued, would need to be

> attentive to people who are left out, e.g., those alienated by religious language, or men who are not involved in religious activity. . . . What that means hasn't been acknowledged or discussed . . . [The] centrality of Gender has popped up but has not been adequately addressed. . . . How will language get in the way of ARHAP making headway in social sciences and public health? The justification of my involvement to my colleagues may be difficult. Other individuals and professionals may not be as forgiving as me.[82]

Despite immense efforts by the consortium's researchers, including a strong theoretical foundation, it is still today not entirely clear that ARHAP-related activities have countered these concerns in a way that would reassure skeptical outsiders. The majority of researchers are identified with traditional Christianity, but also do manifest diversity: ranging from American evangelicals engaged in traditional medical missions, to alternative health workers such as Dr. Jo Wreford, a white South African anthropologist who also practices folk medicine as an *isangoma* and explores what she called "the discomfiting question of witchcraft discourse."[83] Still, one wonders what the Memphis model might look like outside the Bible Belt, for example, in a religiously diverse city like San Francisco, Boston, or London.

Scorgie's comments about homogeneity also highlight a troubling concern about the racial balance of the research teams, particularly as they are reflected in leadership roles. Despite its focus on health equity for poor black persons in Sub-Saharan Africa and select communities in the American South, there is no getting past the fact that most authors on key ARHAP literature, and all of the lead authors, are white. This disparity is particularly stark in the context of South Africa and against the background of a consortium that has historically drawn from a very strong anti-apartheid vision. This apparent leadership disparity is certainly *not* intentional; it is also very clear that black individuals have been actively involved from the beginning as vibrant players in leading the service programs (for example in the Memphis CHN and the Masangane program in South Africa, where the founders and original clergy leaders were also women), as coauthors on a number of papers, and as graduate students, including those who served as mentors across the Atlantic, from South Africa to the United States, to provide advice and guidance on shaping asset-based programs for health in the American South. The appearance of a deficit in black leadership of ARHAP may in part point to a broader and more fundamental tragedy—in any society and group, religious or not—of historical trends that risk perpetuating inequities in health, economics, education, and ultimately leadership and an affirmation of agency and creative potential in a community to make real change possible. To their credit, ARHAP researchers and practitioners clearly recognize this concern.

The ARHAP model is also not (or not overtly) a human rights–based approach to health (see Chapter 4). Even though clear legal covenants and mandates exist that relate to human rights and health rights in both the United States and South

Africa following apartheid, the ARHAP material for the most part hardly touches on such issues. Such a silence is not unusual, since religious studies scholars are rarely trained in human rights law. And it is quite clear that ARHAP researchers are not against human rights. Any broader application of ARHAP's general conceptual approach would be very compatible with a more intentional engagement in human rights, and both Cochrane and de Gruchy's backgrounds in social activism reflect a strong commitment to justice and the value of championing a legal equity that is directly relevant to economic, social, and cultural rights.[84] In fact, Cochrane notes that, provided it included an element of mutual accountability and obligation, he and de Gruchy conditionally supported a rights-based approach—within certain critical limits:

> For example, we agree(d) with the general African critique of the international instruments as wholly missing the importance of 'obligations' in asserting 'rights.' I would mean here (not speaking for Steve) that our rights are not simply entitlements, but also require of us a striving for the rights of all as an obligation placed upon us if we are to claim any rights at all.[85]

CONCLUSION: A CALL TO RESPECTFUL DIALOGUE

In conclusion, despite these limitations and challenges, ARHAP's consistent emphasis on dialogue and listening remains positive and hopeful. It resonates as a key message that both faith-based and public health groups need to hear as they seek to work together.

Steve de Gruchy summarized this "call to respectful dialogue" in 2007, in a discussion of the basic principles he considered necessary to reach across these interdisciplinary spaces.[86] While his comments, summarized below, focused on work in

Africa, they could also be applicable to any community context where faith-based actors and public health workers coexist and care about health and health conditions.

Public health professionals, he said, must address four challenges if they want to take religion seriously in a dialogue. They must acknowledge the ubiquity of religion in the healthworlds where they work; They must appreciate the convergences, that is, how religious entities are important allies for public health; They must "discover the categories"—the dialogue necessary to learn from each others' differences; And they must "enlarge the table"—to enable all who might have a vital contribution to join the discussion on public health policy and action.

Persons who represent religious positions in such dialogue, he continued, are also responsible for certain challenges. Given the ubiquity of religion, they must accept the responsibility to act in society through public health tasks. It is not enough for them, in his view, to simply provide and support compassionate care for the sick—they must also address preventive issues like clean water, sanitation, nutrition, hygiene, sexual health, reproductive health, and mental health. Like public health experts, religious actors must also embrace the convergences, respecting others they might not agree with, those who also care about well-being within the society. They must be ready and willing to "translate" their own concepts, since religious talk can sometimes come across as "in-speak" or even incomprehensible code words. They must work to ensure that the meaning of what they say is transparent to those in public health and that it allows open, respectful conversation with health partners outside one's own faith circle. Religious actors also need to "value the medics," de Gruchy insisted. Rather than polarizing religious healing practices against the "other" medicine that builds on science, community healing and cross-disciplinary constructive dialogue is possible only when religious actors can also respect the scientific peer-review process, for example, in order to support the "best that both can offer."

Finally, both religious individuals and public health workers share four challenges that confront both groups. Working together will be effective only when they: dialogue with humility; respect the elders—that is, reflecting on the past and what can be learned from it; build capacity so the next generation can take up an ongoing work; and finally, forge solidarity.

Such a dialogue, de Gruchy concluded, "is not about conversation but about transformation. . . . The symbolic vision and calling of religions to transform this world into a better one [and] the commitment of public health to create the conditions where this is possible."

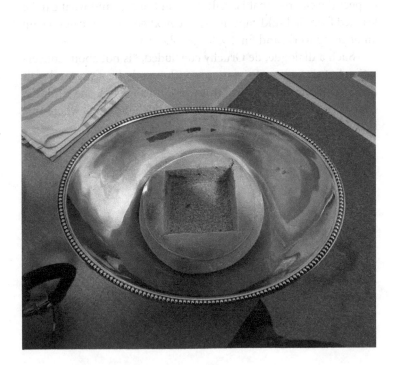

DON'T TEACH ME TO FISH

What's Wrong with Gift-Charity?

IN JANUARY 2010, a few days after the earthquake that destroyed much of Haiti, a "Democracy Now!" news video caught on film a missionary-sponsored helicopter dropping loaves of bread from the air onto the grieving Haitian community in the town of Léogâne. The helicopter had in fact been on the ground a few minutes earlier, then took off and rose to hover several hundred feet above the rubble purposely for the bread "distribution." The aerial donation was completely impersonal, its plastic-encased food raining down as if from a visiting spaceship from another planet.

The Haitian community responded to the bread drop with outrage. As one young man told reporters, "They should have given [it] to the responsible on the ground to distribute to the rest of the people here, and not when they go back up in the air, throw the bread out like they were throwing bones to dogs."[1] Léogâne's mayor, Santos Alexis, sitting in the backyard of the local police station amidst the stench of rotting corpses trapped under the rubble around him, identified the helicopter with an American institution, "you know, a church." He told reporters that the weirdly impersonal donation made his now-homeless constituency "feel humiliated . . . very embarrassed."[2] The event amused and shocked the press, which, with the local community, pointed to it as an example of everything that is wrong in religious attempts at social relief. Instead of mutual respect and intentional conversation between the helicopter's American missionary sponsors and Léogâne's profoundly wounded, hungry, and thirsty human beings, the interchange compounded their victimization with a dehumanizing and humiliating rain of bread from the sky.

Mario Joseph, Haiti's most influential and respected human rights lawyer, reflected on the incident again two years later, as much of the displaced population in Haiti was still struggling to survive in camps. Summarizing the problems with so-called "gifts," he identified issues that are directly relevant to the themes explored throughout this book and his comments are worth quoting here in full:

> [I]t was a missionary helicopter and they had bread. Instead of asking people how to organize to distribute the bread they hovered over the area and just dropped the bread down. It was something that really hurt me. And it really hurt everyone in the area. That's an example that's indicative or really explains all of the aid distribution in Haiti. They never want to plan; for instance if they want to help the people in the camps, they don't sit with the people in the camps to ask how to help them. . . . So what they do is they come with just a little bit. But they come with cameras, and their video cameras to show that they're giving the aid, but it's just a little bit, it's not even a lot. And then you know there are people that are hungry and thirsty, and they fight amongst themselves for the aid. They don't have any choice. That means handicapped people can't get first aid. And people who don't have the will to fight have no access. I don't understand how these civilized countries that say they want to help . . . in distributing aid they need to recognize [people's] rights and dignity.[3]

In the world of faith-based aid related to health, missionary activities, charity, or so-called gifts like the bread drop are what most of us may think of first. In fact, whenever I speak of my work as engaging with the history of faith-based responses to poverty, hunger, and disease, people often assume that this means a focus on handouts, rather than a more nuanced exploration of attitudes and meaning across languages, cultures, and history.

But what is a gift? What does it mean to help another person in a way that promotes individual and community health, including respect for basic human dignity and rights through the exchange of some tangible substance that is (at some level) seen as free? Acts of voluntary, non-economic exchange, whether mutual or one-sided, are all too often, even with the best intentions, plagued by self-interest, the politics of religious power, and rapid emotional burnout of unprotected, naïve and woefully unprepared volunteerism and gender blindness. Donors are frequently acting on deep-seated control issues that keep them from being equally vulnerable to receive anything back, so focused on "doing good" or "helping out" that they may demonstrate insensitivity or blindness to their own and others' real needs, limitations, and equal humanity. I know; I too have done it. And religious groups are often the worst offenders. But does this mean gifts are wrong?

C. S. Lewis captured this tension well in a radio talk on "The Four Loves" in 1958, where he said:

> To receive love that is purely a gift, that bears witness solely to the loving-kindness of the giver, and not at all to our loveliness, is a severe mortification. . . . 'I don't want any of your darned Christian charity' is a very familiar sentence. Of course, it often springs from an ignorance of what Christian charity is, more often from a well-grounded suspicion that Christian charity is not what we are really being offered, because of course much that is called charity contains so much vanity, self-applause, and veiled contempt that it cannot but be resented. It is hard to bear *agape* from our fellows. And yet each of us needs it.[4]

This chapter is—very intentionally—the only one in this book that focuses even obliquely on what might be traditionally called religious charity. In all my writing on faith-based responses to poverty in Christian history, I have tried very hard to avoid the term charity, since I generally believe that this word—like the word love—is often used so broadly that it is functionally meaningless and certainly unhelpful in any discussion about what is good for human beings who suffer the effects of poverty, illness, sorrow, pain, hunger, and injustice in our world.

My concern throughout this book, therefore, is not for almsgiving or philanthropy in general, but only with the conceptual potential of related non-market-based intersections of exchange that address or occur within settings of social poverty and inequity. Charity is often conflated with gift, but in this chapter I suggest they are not quite the same thing. As we know from authors like anthropologist Marcel Mauss and Mary Douglas, as well as social historians like Margaret Visser through her wonderful book, *The Gift of Thanks,* it is possible to receive a gift without it being regarded as charity.[5] What can we learn about the role of the gift in settings where need is more obvious? This chapter will explore this question by reflecting principally on several common contexts for gift exchange that have a particular focus on health, and through a lens that focuses on two basic elements common to such gifts: food and water.

GLOBAL HEALTH AND THE GIFT

As basic elements for life, food and water are often where our gifts to one another begin. Food distribution, rights to food and water, and the global challenge to keep water safe and food healthy shape debates, tensions, and gifts within family and friend dynamics, school breakfast programs, corporate food donations to homeless shelters and food banks, farm subsidies, humanitarian aid, border-control regulations, and global and national health policies. Spoilage and contamination, theft, and corruption related to food supplies and distribution are common risks. Food and water are also metaphors for other types of charitable gift dynamics. Their deep cultural meanings and uses in ritual and feast emphasize that faith-based gift exchanges for health (whether the exchange is one-sided or both parties give *and* receive) require far more than mere fulfillment of basic bodily needs. Pilgrims to the Kumbh Mela, described in Chapter 2, often take home a bottle of Ganges river water; and blessed water—whether from the Jordan River or the bathroom tap with an added ritual blessing—is often also sprinkled or distributed (usually both) in Christian liturgical practices. To give and exchange food and water sufficient for community and global health invites an attitude of mindfulness about the whole person—not merely their minimum daily requirements, but a cultural adequacy for human flourishing. To consider gift-charity through a focus on food and water also evokes the tensions of essential reciprocity. While it may be easy for me to mail a gift of money to a distant land, empowering others to adequate food and water tends, more often than not, to invite me to get personal about the exchange: to share a meal, even to risk taking into myself the true kindness and gentle generous goodness of someone else's cooking and to defer to others when it comes to the hygiene of their eating utensils. We may all know people who use food and water access as a means for power control (their own or others'). More constructively, however, activities that engage us with justice related to global and individual food and water adequacy may include community-based social practices that make us vulnerable as recipients. This was the dilemma of Joseph Lumbard (described in Chapter 2), when he chose to accept the hospitality of a cup of water that he correctly suspected would make him very sick. Whether we ourselves would make a similar choice is a deeply personal decision, based on our own health histories and needs. It may well be that a prudent deliberation to practice such openness as Lumbard's in certain circumstances is, at least philosophically, a good thing. It reminds us that we are not alone, and that we cannot change the world all by ourselves. Whether we share the food and water of others or abstain due to well-founded concerns about sanitation and health, such a call to receptivity from the other communicates a truth: that we are all interdependent; we need the healthy support of one another.

Giving anything—including food and water—also mandates respect and support for the agency of the other person: that is, their legitimate option to receive or reject as active agents, to make choices about what is best in their context and culture about what they receive and what they may offer in return. This matters, said South African theologian Steve de Gruchy, because "the very act of compromising the agency and assets [of the poor] is itself an act of injustice."[6] Faith-based gift exchange that promotes global health must begin with donors (or mutual partners in an exchange) who willingly choose to face risks inherent in reciprocity and return; that which we get back may be unpredictable indeed.

Let us look at what this can mean in three interpretive contexts: first, the popular food proverb about "teaching to fish" as it relates to *economic development*, in an example from Malawi and a story about gift aid from Zambia; second, liturgy and historical images of *gratitude and blessing*; and third, the differences, gift ideas, and tensions in the contrast between humanitarian relief and *building solidarity* assets. The chapter concludes the book with some brief thoughts on what such gift dynamics may mean, particularly within the Christian tradition, in how we might think creatively and fairly about our own "beholdenness" in faith-based social action.

GIVE A MAN A FISH . . . ?

A few years ago, I was invited to speak at a religious conference that was debating various perspectives on the popular—and probably ancient Confucian—proverb, "Give a man a fish and he will eat for a day; teach him to fish and he will eat for a lifetime." This proverb is commonly cited in debates over economic development programs for communities marked by poverty. It is sometimes used when the speaker hopes to "prove" that unconditional gifts are wrong, or to defend limitations on personal, church, or government support. Those who appeal to this proverb may suggest that education or skills training are all that we need to become successfully self-sufficient. In the end I was unable to accept the invitation, but the conference title got me thinking about why this issue—and this proverb—are so very controversial.

The "gospel of self-sufficiency," the idea that teaching people to help themselves is all that really matters in poverty relief, has never made sense to me. This may be because I began my professional life working as a registered dietitian and public health nutrition educator in a government food program that recognized the value of both teaching and giving at the same time. While this program is by no means perfect, it remains an instructive example of how improving the agency (that is, the ability to make their own decisions and act on them) of individuals, in this case mothers, in any household can improve the health of an entire community.

I was working in the Women, Infants, and Children (WIC) Supplemental Food Program.[7] Established in 1972, WIC both *gives* and *teaches*. Pregnant and breastfeeding women and mothers of children with an eligible health-related risk (for example, anemia, obesity, underweight, or short stature) are required to meet for a (free) personal consult with a trained nutrition educator (such as a registered dietitian) at least once every six months, in a discussion that can help personalize the program's benefits to their or their child's specific needs and cultural preferences. WIC is also about "giving away food," issuing vouchers valid only for very specific (free) groceries that promote health and contain essential nutrients. WIC is emphatically *not* welfare, and it is often tragic to see the palpable shame of women in the grocery store checkout who need to keep these foods separate and explain them to the cashiers while other customers roll their eyes and whisper "food stamps" to other impatient shoppers. WIC is not food stamps. As a government program, it also has no religious component, although recipients typically choose and use the food options according to their culture and faith beliefs. The program's local nature in community health centers also fosters informal relationships and friendships that frequently include conversations about religious beliefs and practices. WIC is not perfect; its funding has been systematically slashed by one presidential administration after another and is now a mere shadow of the original vision to support the health and developmental potential of children in America. But its effectiveness rests on both its free gifts and its teaching components of interactive dialogue with individuals at risk in the local community setting. Its tight administrative constraints minimize the risks of corruption and program abuse, and WIC puts power firmly in the hands of women. It is women who, studies have shown, are most likely to make the greatest difference in children's health and ensure that resources actually and fully benefit the children they are meant for.[8]

Self-sufficiency can of course be very good. It is certainly a vital part of acting as a mature adult. But learning is an ongoing process, and gaining life skills often requires give and take. The focus on capacity building in the "give a fish" proverb seems to overlook some of the economic, cultural, and even religious issues that may present insurmountable obstacles. For example—just to play devil's advocate with the image of fishing—what if you are the man or woman who needs help and your fishing teacher is an outsider to your culture who has flown into your village to try to force you to follow his or her very different way of thinking? What if the hungry person is allergic to fish? What if the fish in the only available streams are polluted by industrial mercury or other toxic wastes? What if the only person in town with power over fishing rods and water rights will (after the teacher finally goes home) make such employment difficult or impossible, or demand a large percentage of your profit? What if the hungry person is a woman who must depend on an abusive partner for the cutting instruments to clean and bone the fish she catches? What if she (or he) must depend on someone else who will demand and abuse the market profits? In short, skill building is only one very small fleck of paint in a vastly broader canvas of interactions that can (but might not) help to promote global health through empowering people to be sufficient and self-motivated agents of their own resources and choices.

Sociologists and anthropologists Ann Swidler and Susan Cotts Watkins identified such challenges more specifically in a 2009 study, "'Teach a man to fish': The sustainability doctrine and its social consequences."[9] Their research was based on years of learning from communities in Malawi, a very poor nation in Africa that ranks near the bottom of the "Human Development Index."

Swidler and Watkins knew from experience that most NGOs who were funding innovative development efforts operated by inviting groups to compete for grants through proposals that presented fundable ideas according to specific rules. The administration, funding, and eligibility criteria of such grants were (and this is common in many other places too) usually based in a wealthy Western nation; those who judge the funding applications, that is, are rarely native citizens of the country or culture where the applicants live and where the intended project will take place. This difference fosters a model of patronage that creates invisible barriers between donor and recipients. Donors usually want quick results so they can report "success" to their supporters, often limiting the grant period to a one-to-three-year cycle. They favor start-ups or short-term projects and almost never promise continuity beyond the initial cycle; even if a funder promises support for many years with the best of intentions, this may not happen. Funds can dry up and disappear and promises can be broken. Such a time-limited and resource-limited approach has created major challenges, for example, in health-care delivery programs for HIV/AIDS. If you want to start someone on antiretroviral (ARV) therapy, and you cannot guarantee—and deliver—lifelong access to the affordable drugs they need for healthy survival, you (and they) face a much-debated serious moral and ethical quandary that has a direct impact on their quality of life and survival.

Partly to avoid such empty promises, development efforts since the late 1990s have sometimes incorporated "asset-based" development approaches (described in Chapter 5). The goal of an asset-based action plan is ideally to support the power of the poor community or individuals who want help to develop community-based and community-directed innovative ideas that will draw on resources that they already have. What Swidler and Watkins saw happening was, rather, a profoundly disempowering application of this idea that was actually causing great harm in its social consequences, by using the "assets" idea as an excuse not to fund essential resources like food, water, and drugs in the grants they offered. Instead, grant applicants were competing for funds that would limit them to spending resources only on training sessions, discussion and evaluation groups, and the creation of ideas. Such talking groups were not helping the people who needed it most. To learn more about why the model didn't work, the two anthropologists interviewed hundreds of local people in Malawi to hear what they thought would work better. Their findings are important because they reflect very common practices in many other communities, including those funded and directed by religious organizations.

What Malawians told them pointed to a long history of disconnect between donors' attitudes and the actual realities of poverty and need. Local applicants in fact worked very hard to get what funding was available, but honing their skills at grant-writing seemed to result in a vicious cycle that, Swidler and Watkins saw, offered "intelligent, educated locals only years of insecure work as 'volunteers,' punctuated by occasional access to 'training' in knowledge and skills that are often irrelevant." Although most funding opportunities were aimed at creating "autonomy, empowerment, self-reliance, and a coherent rational modernity," in fact, "the *actual practices* dictated by the sustainability doctrine have created nearly its opposite." The young bright applicants—who were literate and perceptive enough to know how to play the system and win—saw these monies as a sort of "glittering castle," a promise out of poverty that led instead to perpetual frustration. The promised opportunities fed their hopes for an exit out of village poverty rather than a chance to strengthen the health of the village and themselves within it. Given the local and national job markets, often their highest imaginable goal was a job in the administrative strata of one of these aid organizations, perpetuating the very programs that were not effecting positive change where it mattered in their country. Such jobs hardly nurtured "sustainable" health; instead they enabled perpetuating dysfunction.

The Malawi applicants sometimes tried to make the funds work where it would count. In writing proposals, they told Swidler and Watkins, the local leaders strategized about "ways to camouflage what they really need—support for the elderly, the poor, children, and the ill; agricultural inputs like fertilizer or breeding hens; blankets and school uniforms. . . . [V]illagers do know what they want but little of it is training [for things that] they already know how to do." In sum, the researchers concluded, the ideal of sustainability as it is usually understood through the "teaching to fish" model is "a convenient self-delusion for funders."

These findings should matter to anyone who works in faith-based dialogue about poverty, especially those of us conditioned to think skeptically about the value of free handouts. If Swidler and Watkins are right, and the dominant model today does not work where it matters most, then we in the funding-rich West need to stop forcing funds onto this model and focus instead on what really does foster sustainable global health and human potential. We may also need to face the fact that, as Buddhist writer David Loy put it, "The dismal record of the last 50 years of development reveals the cruelty of the usual slogan: when we have taught the world's poor to fish, the effect has often been to deplete their fishing grounds for our consumption."[10]

What is important here is not to criticize what goes wrong, but to reflect on how gifting may play a role in opportunities and activities that can succeed in improving global health. We can learn about examples of good outcomes, for instance, from organizations such as the Abdul Latif Jameel Poverty Action Lab at the Massachusetts Institute of Technology; studies like *Portfolios of the Poor*,[11] the World Bank's three-volume series, *Voices of the Poor*;[12] the "Millions Saved" case studies from the "What Works Working Group" in the Washington DC–based Center for Global Development;[13] or watchdog economic monitors like Transparency International.[14]

Whether we belong to a faith community or not, it is often too easy to condemn religious activities just because we personally may not agree with their teachings or because we hear about encounters like the Haiti missionary bread drop. No response to human need is an instant fix-it. Most of the good examples depend on complex dynamics by imperfect people whose work weaves connective threads across and within entire communities in relationships of trust and effective respect, dignity, and honest communication. Such relationships are never easy or simple.

HAVE YOU EATEN ANYTHING?

This chapter opened with a story of food aid that illustrated a shameless and inexplicable violation of basic human dignity and respect following the 2010 earthquake in Haiti. The research from Malawi shows how development grants also fail to get at what people may really need for a just approach to health. Another story, from Zambia, may suggest a more encouraging model of faith-based food gifts based on very small-scale solidarity, although this example too is not without challenges.

Zambia is, like Malawi, a poor country in Sub-Saharan Africa. In April of 2005, three researchers for the African Religious Health Assets Programme (described in Chapter 5) visited the community of Bauleni in the province of Lusaka as part of a "participatory inquiry," a quest to learn if and why religion made any difference in the way people thought about health. The team was directed by Steve de Gruchy, a native of South Africa and professor of religion and theology at the University of KwaZulu-Natal in Pietermaritzburg. Working with de Gruchy were two of his graduate student researchers, Sinatra Matimelo, a pastor and former banker from Zambia, and the Rev. Mary Mwiche.

The team walked through the village, asking questions, and met with several groups to listen and record community narratives about health, religion, and healing. At the Bauleni Pentecostal Church they heard this story:

> As a pastor, we had a patient who was sick, a church member, and we prayed for her for two weeks, and each time there was no improvement. Until one time the spirit of God says, 'can you just ask, if she has eaten anything?' So I asked, 'Madam, have you eaten anything?' And she said, 'how can I get anything?' So the church decided to do something. In the afternoon they all went and bought her this and that, such as a bag of maize-meal. And the very next morning . . . she was healed![15]

This deceptively simple tale illustrates several key points about charity and gift that have been explored in this chapter. The speaker is a pastor who is part of the local community, remembering an encounter with a woman who everyone in the room (except the researchers) would have known. This woman had turned to the church for the only solution she could count on: prayer. Pentecostal Christians take prayer very seriously; it must have been hard for the pastor to admit that prayer had not worked for this woman, not because she did anything wrong, but simply because she needed something else: something as "worldly" as food. Prayer led to a divine "nudge," and thanks to the spirit of God, someone thought to ask, "Has she eaten?" Hunger was so normal for this woman (and presumably those in her church) that—for two weeks, it appears—no one happened to notice that she was starving. But as soon as the suggestion went public, the church community mobilized their resources, their internal assets, into action.

Like de Gruchy and his listening team, we, too, know nothing, really, about why this woman was sick, or if her "healing" would hold up under evidence-based medical scrutiny. But we do know how hunger works. We know that her likely chronic hunger and related malnutrition had reduced her immune system's ability to fight disease, making it more likely that she could die from even a simple illness.[16] A 2012 Food and Agricultural Organization (FAO) report on the *State of Food Insecurity in the World* today has estimated that about 870 million people remain chronically malnourished, with about 850 million of them living in developing countries.[17] We know that she was a poor woman in a poor country who had likely very poor sanitation and also likely lacked reliable access to clean water. Basic hygiene, sanitation, and clean water are low-cost solutions that can make a big difference to health.[18] We also know that her chronic starvation would have made it harder for her to bounce back or have energy for work (if work was available), since the starving body makes it hard to focus, learn, and find the energy to act or realize one's potential, perpetuating chronic inequities.

We might also wonder why the church needed "the spirit of God" to see that she was starving. But poverty and hunger are so common in many places that they can be all but invisible. And women traditionally get shortchanged on food in many cultures. In Sub-Saharan Africa today, it is estimated that more than a quarter of the entire population is undernourished; this situation was far worse in Zambia in 2005, when it was estimated that 71 percent of Zambians lived in "abject poverty."[19] This hungry woman's church could afford to pray, but providing food called for gathering sacrificial portions of "this and that." Development programs like those in Swidler and Watkins's Malawi—if they even existed in this woman's community—would not have provided food, and would more likely have caused a church's brightest and most promising youth to leave town to learn to write grant applications. De Gruchy and his researchers might be suspected of having time for their research thanks to exactly one of these sorts of grants that focus on gathering information rather than on direct provision of food, medicine, or other resources; but the problem Swidler and Watkins described is not that such grants exist, but that too often they offer the only options for communities in need. Unfortunately, even multinational secular NGOs who do provide medicines—and who bring innovative health care and health-care delivery methods to poor communities—rarely include food and nutrition in essential health-care services. Why should we expect faith communities to be different?

LITURGICAL GIFTS: OF GRATITUDE AND BLESSING

Food and water—the very substances excluded from the common development grant model and essential for the woman's survival in Zambia—are also central in the role of the gift in religious liturgy. Such liturgies touch on gifting relevant to poverty, but cannot be reduced to "charity." The liturgical reciprocity of gift *exchange* dominates early Christian and Jewish texts. A key element in such practices is the concept of *gratitude*. But if social justice is about helping people realize their *entitlements,* what does it mean to say "thank you"?

In anthropology, and sometimes also in religious practice, a "pure gift" is generally understood as an exchange free of any self-interest, an offering that expects no compensation from the recipient. But this idea is a messy one in religion, where it is often claimed simultaneously with a teaching that one will indeed receive a reward—from God—if perhaps not in this present life. The religious idea of the pure or free gift to benefit the poor is not limited to monotheistic religions. In India, a similar concept is that of *dan,* which in Hinduism signifies "a gift offered through desireless action."[20] Ideally described as giving "in order to forget," *dan* has, like Western alms, come to encompass a broad range of donations for the poor that don't necessarily fit a strictly selfless image.

"There should not be any free gifts," said anthropologist Mary Douglas. By this she meant that when such so-called pure gifts are seen as charity they wound the poor by aggravating the tensions of social inequality, undermining human dignity, and fostering dependence. In such experiences, as also in Douglas's experience working for a charitable foundation, "the recipient does not like the giver, however cheerful he be."[21] And indeed the shame and stigma of poverty, including the shame of being an object of charity, handicaps many, who then experience a lifelong struggle with low self-esteem, a deep sense of inferiority, and an inability to take themselves seriously enough to pursue with confidence ambitions that in fact they are often capable of attaining successfully.

This disempowerment of shame also crosses generations, affecting children as they inhabit the effects of their parents' economic fears. I remember how angry my mother would sometimes get when my brother or I got sick or hurt ourselves badly enough to need medical attention. Part of her anger was rooted in her own extreme childhood poverty, her response to a deprivation that had enabled her to save face by denying any need for charity. To see her children in pain, I think, cracked that defense in a way that made her angry precisely because, as we knew well, she did love us very much. But her anger—which came across to me at least as a message of blame and shame—was also triggered by something much more straightforward: health insurance coverage. Although both parents were working, we survived on very spare resources, and the only health insurance available through my father's employer required a hefty deductible up front at every medical visit, a deductible that our parents could barely afford. For years I internalized my mother's fearful anger so well that it sometimes seemed easier to live with the pain of an injury or illness rather than risk her attention by admitting a need for medical help. For me as a child, therefore, health care seemed at best a costly charity. Happily, we were for the most part healthy kids who also (ironically enough) lived in a region known for some of the best and most abundant health-care resources in America. We always received the treatment we needed—eventually. But these experiences were a deep lesson in the limits of private medical insurance in the United States and the vital importance of prompt treatment and adequate coverage for all as essential in truly global health. Millions around the world live (and die) in circumstances where they lack access to even the most basic medical resources that might be practically available to themselves, their family, or their community. If charity merely perpetuates social and economic injustice, it is right, I believe, to be angry at the system, but not at those (adults or children) whose very ordinary human vulnerabilities deserve the dignity of decent care.

There are two popular—and vastly different—views in modern American society on why free gifts are seen as wrong. One view—that of those who are often called economic and political conservatives—argues against handouts because, so they say, the poor should be made to work for whatever they get. This is a variant of the opinion that charity hurts the *donor*, that is, by wasting his or her money on a scheme that undercuts the social muscle of a capitalist society where human value is measured by work and production. The second view—the opinion of Mary Douglas and Haiti's human rights lawyer quoted earlier, and held by many so-called political and economic liberals—argues that, in contrast, such one-sided free handouts hurt the *recipients*. In this view, those who receive are hurt by a donation that deprives them of something far more important than economic performance: the respect they deserve from others on the basis of their agency and personhood as human beings who by nature are created to engage in social and material *reciprocity*. In other words, both conservatives and liberals actually agree that so-called free handouts for the poor are problematic. They differ, however, in their view of who gets hurt, what to do about it, and why. And if charity is sanctioned in certain settings, there may be disagreement on the value of the gift, the value of the other person, and the relative value of the donor's time and resources.

But what of the moral value for gratitude? The dynamics of gratitude are complex. The Russian poet Marina Tsvetaeva, who survived by living in an unheated room with her two children on the charity of friends when she was oppressed by ruling Bolshevists soon after the 1917 Russian Revolution, could not bring herself to thank her friends. Ashamed by the unequal power relationship of alms from friends, she felt that saying "thank you" would be a degeneration into "paid love . . . an outright offense to the giver as well as the recipient . . . and an obstacle to the development of lasting ties."[22] She chose, she wrote, an intentionally "silent gratitude" as the only acceptable response. Others may attempt to cope with the shame of charity by using it to help those around them. I once had an aunt who gladly accepted all the government-surplus food she could get (and was qualified for)—and then gave our family what she didn't want. For many years growing up, the little that I knew about government aid to the poor in America was poignantly symbolized by a couple of irrelevant heavy glass bottles of Karo syrup that sat gathering dust in the back of a bottom cupboard. Still others may handle the indignities of dehumanizing shame by condemning the donors. The Haitian citizens of Léogâne, whose story opens this chapter, felt that the helicopter bread drop called for public rage. "This is pure humiliation," said one young man in Haiti who had spent the previous week organizing his neighborhood to dig bodies from the rubble; "We don't want their stinking bread."[23]

Marcel Mauss's classic study on *The Gift*—and much recent anthropology as well—does not focus principally on help for the poor. And few of the other recent studies on social gift exchange and gratitude[24] consider faith-based aid. We find an exception in essays by several historians who have recently published on the concept of the gift in antiquity.

In one study, historian Gregg Gardner looked at early rabbinic Jewish ideas of gifts to the poor that help mitigate the "wounding" effect of one-sided charity.[25] The rabbis in late antiquity, Gardner noted, knew all about this troubling paradox of hurtful gifting and the need for corrective dignity and justice. They addressed the problem by hedging gifts theologically with language of reciprocity. Changing the conceptual understanding of a gift into one that carried a meaning of reciprocal exchange (as a "loan," for example) was necessary precisely because in Judaism *charity*—tzedakah—was a moral mandate. Another scholar, Tzvi Novick, explored how gift-giving rules for Purim in Palestinian rabbinic sources blunt the social distinctions between tzedakah and the idea of "reciprocation of kindness."[26]

In several recent studies, historian Daniel Caner has focused on the detailed nuances of alms, blessings, and offerings in sixth- and seventh-century Christianity. While gift-charity and social justice are sometimes polarized in dialogue about aid, early Christian texts from late antiquity also interweave these ideas together with gifting.[27] Tzedakah, for example, meant both alms and righteousness to late-antique Jews as well as Syriac-speaking Christians such as Rabbula of Edessa, a fifth-century bishop active in health-care reform, the establishment of free hospitals, and details such as sanitation and the role of hospital attendants for the poor sick.[28] Indeed, true social justice in many biblical and patristic texts is understood as demanding an inseparable application of both justice *and* mercy, and this package of pre-scribed behaviors manifested "righteousness" as well as "loving kindness." Such close conceptual pairing is so tightly integrated in the modern Christian tradition that the late Krister Stendahl, Lutheran bishop of Stockholm and a forthright voice in global ecumenical dialogue, wrote,

> The basic point is that we should not think of judgment and
> mercy as two different things, . . . Judgment is mercy for those
> who need mercy. Judgment is justice for those who hunger
> and thirst after it, since they do not have it. . . . In the world
> one speaks about justice and in the church one speaks about

righteousness. But Hebrew, Greek, and Latin do not offer this distinction.[29]

Gratitude was an important part of these expectations for the poor in the early Christian era. We see this at its simplest level in the story of Jesus healing ten lepers in Luke 17:11–19. When only one returned to thank him—to "give praise to God"—Jesus asked, "Where are the other nine?" Sirach 35:4, which many early Christians read as scripture, equates alms with a "thank offering." And 2 Timothy 3:2 closely associates "ungrateful" with "unholy" on a list of the sort of Christians that their fellow believers ought to avoid. Prayer was regarded as a form of gratitude in early Christian texts, where the poor who received aid—especially widows—were perceived as having an obligation to give back to the church by, for example, praying for their benefactors.[30]

Gregory, the Christian bishop of Nazianzus (modern central Turkey) in the fourth century, was also explicit about such gratitude as a moral mandate that had particular importance for the poor. We find this idea in two of his sermons (Orations 19.9 and 24.18), where he argues that *gratitude* is precisely that gift which the poor—who, after all, have nothing else—offer up as their way to honor God, expressing it either directly or through their pious acts of recognition of and honor to the martyrs. In context, Gregory recites a systematic list of who owes what, assigning specific virtuous acts to different ages and genders across the social spectrum according to their role in society; the appropriate moral actions that are suitable gifts from: young women, matrons, young men, old men, civil authorities, military authorities, men of letters, priests, laity, those in mourning, successful men, the rich, and the poor. Both lists conclude by calling for *generosity* from the rich and *gratitude* from the poor, pairing the two phrases in a way that strongly suggests an expected perceived interdependence between them.

Thanksgiving also finds central expression in Christian liturgical practice through the exchange of small tokens known as *eulogiae* (or "blessings"). According to Caner, these were very small gifts distributed by religious leaders to clerics, monks, and pious travelers, including the poor and sick in search of healing and justice.[31] Caner locates the root of this idea in the New Testament, where Paul speaks in 2 Cor. 9:5–12 of the spiritual blessings or enrichment that follows from giving small amounts of extra goods to the poor and to the holy. *Eulogiae* could be tiny pieces of bread, small amounts of money, or some other material substance that was perceived to have a spiritual power to do good. By the fifth and sixth centuries, when this practice found its way into patristic literature, *eulogiae* represented "an early Byzantine example of a pure gift ideal, in the classic sense of a gift that imposed no obligation on its receiver to reciprocate or make a return."[32] Blessings could come from what the faithful offered to God, and they could lead to all (or part) being used in turn for alms for the poor. But blessings were distinct from alms: anyone, poor or rich, could ask for and receive a blessing, while alms, Caner suggests, were exclusively for the poor. The concept of *eulogiae* persists today in extra-eucharistic practices associated with the Christian liturgy of the Orthodox Church, for example, in the practice of "prosphora" bread. After the priest blesses the loaf that will be used for the eucharistic celebration but before it is consecrated, he removes a section of it for the eucharistic consecration, and cuts the remaining unconsecrated loaf (illustrated in the photo that begins this chapter) into small squares that are available for distribution after the eucharist to everyone present, regardless of religious affiliation. Loaves that are designated as *prosphora* are also part of this intentional practice of sharing and generosity. This exchange is often marked by a parity of reciprocity, and portions are sometimes taken home to those who cannot be present for the eucharistic liturgy.

If the key to a health-giving liturgical gift in early Christian sources was in the manner of exchange and social interdependence, it was also shaped by views about relative social status.

Reciprocity between people who are economically and socially "unequal"—such as from the rich to the poor—may not seem like a mutually beneficial exchange. It is a truism that the poor in every culture practice philanthropy among themselves—often more generously than the rich—but, as some anthropologists note, poor individuals who engage in these exchanges may look blank or puzzled if you ask them what they gave back in their aid exchanges with those who are more wealthy or powerful than themselves.[33]

Sociologist LiErin Probasco has recently explored this dynamic and value of liturgical exchanges across cultural and social groups, particularly the role of blessings and gratitude. Probasco's research was based on fieldwork about North American short-term missions projects in Nicaragua.[34] Her informants—Nicaraguan villagers who participated in one of two very different types of faith-based aid initiatives that engaged partners or volunteers from the United States—tended to consistently regard their Western beneficiaries as active and themselves as passive, even when the Nicaraguan informant was obviously (to Probasco, at least) intensely proactive in local community development activities.

Probasco observed the Nicaraguan Christians practicing a high level of reciprocal "giving back." This practice took the shape of symbolic objects and actions offered as "gifts" from poor community villagers in Nicaragua to the short-term missionary workers. She noticed that symbolic activities seemed to take the place of material gifts such as food or drink, often rejected by the American travelers, "not only because of contamination but also because they believed it could not be spared."[35] While religious narratives such as offers of prayer helped bridge this gap, self-perceptions of disparity remained:

> Despite evidence of locally initiated community development projects, the religious language that I heard locals use with foreign donors left little space for collective Nicaraguan moral

agency apart from an all-powerful God, God-appointed foreign emissaries, and devout Nicaraguan recipients.[36]

Probasco advises those who might lead such gift-based mission teams to keep in mind seven key lessons for shaping their dialogue and action. Outside organizations intent on "helping" in such settings should, she suggested: know the community's narrative; connect with long-term programming; practice social reflexivity; educate team members (before they leave home); publically recognize the gifts and contributions of hosts; make the link between global and local; and perform post-travel follow-through to reflect on goals and shape what happens next.[37]

As we may try to tease out whether a particular example of aid is problematic charity, justice, or gift in similar cross-cultural settings today, we may need to ask related questions about our own perceptions, whether we practice philanthropic tourism or not. For example: What exactly is being exchanged? What is the power differential and how does the exchange enact (or not) a healthy life-giving redemptive space for the person who has the greatest material need in this exchange? What is the metaphorical location of donors' and recipients' bodies and faces in such activities: Are they worlds apart, face-to-face, or shoulder-to-shoulder as they walk together? What are the expectations for the exchange? Is the exchange nothing more or less than an employment model, and does it have anything to do with justice? If it seems to be perceived as win-win, how do we know what is win for the other? How does the exchange respect human dignity? And who decides on the gift?

FROM HUMANITARIAN RELIEF TO SOLIDARITY ASSETS

Faith-based food aid as gift operates most acutely today in the realm of humanitarian aid and emergency relief. Disaster relief or humanitarian aid is big business in much of the world. Such emergency aid focuses on saving lives fast by targeting intensive donations that provide food, water, medical care, and housing in highly unstable situations marked by man-made and natural disasters: flood, earthquake, political chaos, and refugee displacement. Such emergency gifts are usually justified by the argument that a particular crisis has made local conditions so severe that cultural sensitivities to empower, accompany, and foster solidarity and sustainability are impractical goals in the urgency to keep people alive this minute.

Crisis settings by their very nature destabilize delivery access and infrastructure, things like storage and refrigeration, and food preparation methods. Charitable shipments to areas of civil strife are often diverted and commandeered by the warring forces of those in power, who may limit distribution to loyal partisans or sell them for weapons or personal luxuries while terrorizing refugees and NGOs who are trying to help.[38] In most settings, all too often, money raised (or promised) from afar rarely seems to reach its targeted use. Emergency *medical* aid is sometimes more consistently hopeful, since it requires the presence of highly skilled health-care workers with a specific purpose. But often even medical aid may "parachute" into an infrastructure that lacks tools that the volunteer doctor may take for granted at home (such as reliable electricity or parts and skills available for repairs and maintenance). Medical groups who address these needs vary in their ethical approach to political neutrality. For example, Médecins sans Frontières/Doctors without Borders (MSF) is committed to "witness" or speak out publically and take a stand on political issues they view as unjust or harmful, while some other international medical aid organizations have a policy of neutrality, helping everyone without distinction between political loyalties or military roles in a particular civil or guerrilla conflict. Policy differences may similarly affect faith-based efforts. Those who choose to get involved should know exactly what they are getting into before they commit themselves, make decisions slowly and carefully, and anticipate clearly in advance the possible consequences and ethics of what they want to do. Unfortunately, such advance planning often seems to be impossible in real life, but the better-prepared and aware one is, the more likely she or he is to be part of a solution rather than perpetuating a chronic injustice or aggravating frustrations. As in other gift-justice actions generally, the most effective actions likely draw on the experience of many years and a long-term, even lifelong, commitment to local relationships of mutual respect.

Dignity and respect sometimes matter even more than necessary food and safe living conditions. Cardinal Francis George, Catholic Archbishop of Chicago, realized this when Mexican agricultural workers living in shacks asked him to help them form a union. He certainly knew from their lives that they desperately needed higher wages and better-insulated houses to protect them from the desert environment where winters could drop to 20 or 30 degrees below zero. But in fact, they told him, their real need for a union was not really related to material goods. "Bishop," they said, "We want a union because the owners don't respect us." In the ensuing dialogue with the owners, the bishop noted, the Mexican workers focused their demands on nuanced cultural changes in how they related to one another.[39] Human dignity in faith-based aid is often far more complex than simple economic adjustment, and is instead deeply tied to solidarity and accompaniment.

Solidarity and accompaniment are ideas central to Catholic Social Thought and liberation theology. Such ideas also inform NGOs that may not be explicitly religious. One example is that of Partners In Health (PIH), founded in the early 1980s by two Harvard physicians and their friends. PIH has as its guiding philosophy "the preferential option for the poor," the view best known in liberation theology that God has a special concern for the poor. Like liberation theology, PIH is not principally about gifts or charity; its focus is on social justice, with a particular emphasis on engaging in solidarity with those who are in need.

In a talk given several months after the Haiti earthquake in 2010, one physician from PIH, Dr. Paul Pierre, who grew up in Haiti and now works in Malawi where he has directed community programs for PIH's sister organization in that country, emphasized the vital importance of reciprocity that builds what he calls "solidarity assets" and "trust assets." In this view, assets, he said, are not so much something that a community already has to help one another (although this too is true); rather, they are intangible tools, qualities, advantages, or gifts that the community chooses to give to those—including outside NGOs and "donor" organizations—who seriously make the commitment to walk alongside and work with them on their own terms. They are assets that potential "donors" need to invest in—seriously, for the long term. Solidarity and trust assets enable effective reciprocity—but they require the transparent integrity of a committed engagement with the community partners. NGOs who want to build such solidarity assets in order to "help," said Pierre, can do it in health-care activities by proving that they can be trusted and relied on, for example, through

> being on time in the clinic, having the drugs there, having a clinician there, having water, having electricity, having internet, providing good services, and [providing] people in those communities who are very, very poor [with] access to those minimum social and economic rights.[40]

BECOMING *EULOGIAE* PEOPLE

Gifts need not be incompatible with solidarity assets in building the healthy community. Ethicist Luke Bretherton has recently explored the language of gift in faith-based civic exchange, in his new book on *Resurrecting Democracy*. Bretherton suggests a gift-based vision of citizenship as part of what he calls "consociational" common life in community. The gift is, he emphasizes, fundamentally a relationship mediated by symbols. In the civic context, gifting matters as it affirms the human social nature of citizenship, because, following Aristotle, "acquisition without reciprocity amounts to acquisition without justice."[41] Gift, he insists, is part of how we relate to one another as human beings, in community and in society. To reject the value of this dynamic is to deny much that is human in social citizenship and honest solidarity. Gifting from one person to another that comes out of twisted motives—to patronize, for example, or somehow "prove" one's ability to be generous with a one-sided push that refuses mutual exchange—is, says Bretherton, a "corruption of grace."

But gift is only one of several kinetic processes that mark the healthy democratic citizenship that is Bretherton's focus. Other "taxonomies of sociology" that must also enter the mix of any truly human and "grace-filled" exchange, he suggests, include: equivalent exchange, redistribution, grace in the deeper religious sense, and communion (or mutual sharing). All of these types of gift relations in sociality, Bretherton argues, "are necessary for human flourishing . . . an absence of one leads to dysfunction in the others."

Gift is often pitted against ideals of equity, but Bretherton's vision for gift woven into the fabric of a civic system is one that is aimed at joyously affirming human diversities in a manner that ultimately affirms human wholeness. Building and sustaining a common life, Bretherton argues, "entails being able to recognize and value the non-equivalence of each person and their unique contributions to the whole." Indeed, he concludes,

> the forms of relation built around gift exchange, grace, and communion . . . are precisely ways of recognizing and valuing persons in non-equivalent ways. So while these forms of relation seem to contradict egalitarian commitments, the paradox is that they are necessary means of upholding and affirming

the genuine equality of each person as a unique and incommensurable human being.

As Bretherton also emphasizes, philanthropy is not the only form of gift relation. Indeed, as many of the stories throughout this book illustrate, the risks and opportunities of global health consist, in essence, of many diverse multidisciplinary and particulate practical responses based on "this and that." Into such a context, small *eulogiae* exchanges—"bite-sized blessings" from across different perspectives, including specializations, skills, applied expertise, gifts, and what some might call "ordinary neighborliness" within and across cultures—might, collectively, have the potential to heal the world.

In Chapter 1, I emphasized that this is not a book about what to do, but rather an exploration of common points of tension at the intersection of religion and health that relate to the interconnections of material exchanges on behalf of those who suffer injustices and inequities wherever they live. As I hope the stories in this book illustrate, a commitment to advance and work for global health requires an integration of many disciplines, attitudes, and actions, drawing on culture and religion as well as human rights, social and economic justice and equity, creative thinking in technology and innovations, and so much more.

Listening to religious history also remains crucial to understanding modern ethics and practice on wealth and poverty. If we want to avoid repeating past disasters and perpetuating what does not work, we need to listen to the voices from other times and cultures and learn how to compare them with voices in our world today. Examples from the past often sound very modern, reminding us that there are no easy answers to these issues.

And yet we may still find ourselves at this point persistently wondering what *we* should do, either as individuals or as community participants within a faith-based setting who wish to nurture global health and respect human rights. How should we act, we

may ask, in the presence of a strong sense of "beholden-ness"—
either our own or that of someone else? If I were pushed to risk a
venture here into prescriptive advice, I would reply to such a question with: It depends. What we might best do depends, I think,
on who *we* are, our opportunities to effect global change, and our
personal "vision of the ought." Whatever we do, we must begin by
learning from and listening to others around us who have far more
and more deeply nuanced wisdom based on a range of encounters,
experiences, and hard lessons in what does and does not help in
these areas. Poverty in any culture is complex, determined by a
nuanced network of individual human need, community dynamics, ethics and dis/respect, systemic errors, injustices, and inequities, as well as a host of other factors. It is not helpful to approach
poverty assuming it is all about money, power dynamics, politics,
sin, greed, or structural violence, though these all contribute. We
need less on "how to fix the problem" and more on accountability
to learn from others across the global setting within this immense
complexity.

The conscientious debates over what to *do* sometimes miss
the obvious truth: we put our words into action all the time.
Every choice we make, whether deliberating about practical ethics or not, illustrates to those around us what we really think and
believe as it relates to that eternal tension of "faith" and "works."
How we relate mind and body will depend on what we think of
the connection between ideas (body, spirit) that can or cannot be
measured, and how we make daily decisions about what is "the
right thing to do." Speaking for and to those who identify with
the Christian tradition, I would say this: If we really believe in the
power of prayer, in the resurrection of the body, in Christ's true
presence in our midst, in the ultimate victory of God's true reality
over the deepest sorrows of life in this world, in the incarnation
of the present moment as something that really matters—if we
truly believe these things, we cannot separate mind and mouth
from the rest of the body. Whatever our faith views, "action" in
response to poverty—whether the poverty is our own, our town's,

our faith community's, or the desperate injustice of a global pattern—is *not* just an external behavior that can be contrasted with talking and thinking. Life is short; let us live out our vocations (whatever they are) by acting with the best holistic integrity that we can manage. Action responding to poverty is not essentially about stuff; it is about how I relate in daily life to everything and everyone that is "other," and how honest I am with myself about the theological integrity of the created world and my place in it.

And when it comes to thinking about those traditional forms of "social action" that commonly define "works," again I would say: the choices we make depend on who we are. Some of us will have the natural gifts, talents, and opportunities to make big changes in global health and human rights practices and policies, to effect "big system" solutions. We may know instinctively when others' advice and warnings to us are nothing more than overcautious and unhelpful attempts to clip our wings and curb our true gifts and vocation. Others of us, like the faith community in the Zambian story, may be among those who live with what seem like crippling inner or circumstantial constraints that force us to work within the context of a more limited focus, creatively altering a few small ideas and actions in everyday life, living in the constant kinetic balance of little blessings, eulogiae of "this and that."

If we think we might be "eulogiae people," cautious but eager to think creatively and push boundaries, we may still feel that we ought to be doing as much as possible to help others in need—and that we ought to be doing it—right now! Those most likely to be reading this particular chapter, I suspect, may, like me, be living with a moral conscience that seems to slip into hyperdrive at inconvenient moments. We may struggle with guilt that we cannot always hear "the spirit of God" even when she is standing on the dirt path in front of us.

Certainly there is a place and need for action; permitting passive victimization is not the route to health, either for ourselves or the world around us. And yet—unless we are emergency physicians trained for such a career—there are also occasions when the most health-giving act in a given situation might be to relax a little and cut ourselves some slack. A decision to act or not in a given encounter with human need is of course an individual choice. But interventions that seem like ways to "help the poor" can also risk doing real (if unanticipated and sometimes unpredictable) damage. This is especially true if we leap into aid or volunteer gifting opportunities that would be better served by a depth of relationship and cultural humility that may take years (or perhaps a lifetime) to develop.

If this is who we are, perhaps we might take to heart the novelist Carlene Bauer's fictionalized advice to an oversensitive poet: "Please do not berate yourself for not inventing the Catholic Worker."[42] Even Dorothy Day, who (with Peter Maurin) invented the Catholic Worker, wrote, "to have undertaken a life of silence, manual labor, and prayer might have been the better way. But I do not know. God gives us our temperaments."[43] Eric Gregory, a political ethicist and religion professor at Princeton, reminds us that the parable of the Good Samaritan was not about saving the world, but about acting ethically in the immediate moment since, after all, "the Samaritan was going down that particular road."[44] And Harvard ethnographer Michael Jackson puts it this way:

> [T]he movement from a local to a global world . . . is as fraught as the journey of life itself. There are always losses as well as gains, and it is never possible to decide in retrospect which of our decisions, or our parents' decisions, were for the best. Rather than strive to do the maximum good, I prefer the Hippocratic principle of doing the least harm . . .[45]

We may need these reminders precisely because modern global health conditions present us with a world where boundaries have collapsed. The human needs of our fellow travelers through life and space are ever present to us and can seem to overwhelm. Our "proximate" daily journeying may bring us alongside needy strangers far outside our culture and front door, yet at the same time "there is no indication that the Good Samaritan spent the rest of his life wandering the byways of ancient Israel looking for remote strangers in need."[46] In a reflection on Luke 14:7–14, in which Jesus tells his followers to make dinner for those who can't reciprocate, historian and writer Lauren Winner puts it this way:

> For many of us in the grocery store, it is relatives—non-cooking spouses, and most especially children—who do not invite us back. . . . So I am going home to cook for my husband and my stepdaughter. I do not have any idea when, or if, or how they might invite me back, or not. But suddenly this very ordinary thing may be a bit of discipleship.[47]

The "glocality" of gift, justice, and health begins with finite exchanges such as this. As Gustavo Gutiérrez reminds us, "finding our own way is the task of our discernment and the goal of our spirituality."[48]

Whatever our gifts and vocation; whatever the examples and stories we find most inspiring: that which helps us face the challenge of each moment's struggle to keep balance may be as simple as staying mindful of what really matters. In the faith tradition that ignites my own vision for meaning, the eternal is about past and future, yes, but it is most crucially manifest in a particular and personal sanctity of an Other effective in, with, and upholding each moment of sacred substance in the here and now. However we each view such cultural and belief systems of others, and their connection—relationships of "beholdenness"—between human rights, honest material needs, potential for health, and grace of our fellow human beings, it seems to me that the essence of effective response in the making of community is not *doing*, but *being*. It is not the stuff we "own," worry about, sort, exchange, and trash, but rather the value of time; not charity, but justice with respect and dignity in all that is both good and intangible in our relationships with one another. This, I suspect, is where life gets real.

ACKNOWLEDGMENTS

The French Dominican Antonin-Gilbert Sertillanges wrote that "every intellectual work begins by a moment of ecstasy."[1] For this book, that moment happened one morning in 2010, on a crowded city bus, while I was working at the François-Xavier Bagnoud (FXB) Center for Health and Human Rights, at Harvard School of Public Health. During my cross-town commute, I entered a sudden moment sharp with perception of the gap between the intense conversations that shaped my thinking on health and human rights and similar—yet also very different—conversations with friends committed to faith-based aid. As the book's focus broadened beyond human rights, I was blessed with the opportunity, in 2011, to join the staff at the Harvard Global Health Institute. For their affirmation and encouragement of my interests across disciplines and across centuries, I thank Dr. Jennifer Leaning, Director of the FXB Center, and Drs. Sue J. Goldie and Glaudine Mtshali, Founding Faculty Director and former Executive Director respectively, of the Harvard Global Health Institute. The ideas expressed in this book have been shaped inevitably by the immense privilege of working with such inspiring leaders, but they do not necessarily reflect either the views of these individuals or those of the Center or the Institute.

For moral and intellectual support on social justice, solidarity, and human rights in practice beginning long before that moment on the bus, I could not have found my way to this project without the collegial friendship of Alec Irwin, Alicia Ely Yamin, Mary Kay Smith Fawzi, Zoe Agoos, Keri Wachter, Monika Szperka, and Drs. Evan Lyon and Paul E. Farmer; as well as Arlan Fuller, Ann Hannum, Curt Peterson, Catlin Rockman, and Tricia Spellman. Harvard School of Public Health Professor Stephen Marks welcomed me as an auditor in his spring course on "World Poverty and Human Rights," lectures that nourished me like essential light and air in a dark time. Dr. Rebecca Weintraub graciously extended me the opportunity to participate in the Global Health Delivery Project's Inaugural Faculty Network in 2012. I also owe thanks to Professor Sumner B. Twiss, then at Brown University, who long ago was the first religion scholar to affirm my curiosity in the history of human rights language in texts from antiquity.

Colleagues from the Seminar on Lived Theology and the University of Virginia have continued to engage as literary conversation partners; for their input on my thoughts about human rights in this book (and the quandary over Henry Trevitt's story), I especially thank Charles Marsh, Chuck Mathewes, John Kiess, Russell Jeung, Shea Tuttle, Alan Jacobs, Carlos Eire, and Mark Gornik. Laura Alexander at UVA stunned me with her perceptive and surprise reading of the human rights chapter. It is also improved (I hope) by thinking through some brief but immensely constructive comments from Stanley Hauerwas; the resulting text should not be taken to reflect his views. On religious influence in the history of the UDHR, Hilary Sherratt Yancey engaged me in one of the most invigorating after-church coffee hours I had in many months, and shared with me her honors thesis on Jacques Maritain; she gives me hope for the future.

Graduate students in a 2012 January term course I taught at Episcopal Divinity School helped me talk through initial ideas on several chapters, and inspired me with their dedication to social justice, human rights, disability rights, ministry, and health. I thank Academic Dean, Angela Bauer-Levesque, and Professor Larry Wills for making that opportunity possible.

In researching the African Religious Health Assets Programme (ARHAP), I was keenly aware of the risk—more like sheer folly—of writing about an active group that I have never met, one deeply shaped by the politics and church history of a country (South Africa) I have never visited. I especially thank three of the collaborative's research leaders, James R. Cochrane, Jill Olivier, and Teresa Cutts, for their grace in commenting on early drafts and especially for their generosity of spirit as they set this interloper straight with true collegial encouragement. Any remaining errors are mine alone.

For grounding, encouragement, and practical assistance in support of my research and travel to India as part of the 2013 Harvard University "Mapping the Kumbh Mela" project, I thank Dr. Sue J. Goldie (again) as well as Meena Hewett, Executive Director of the Harvard University South Asia Institute, and Amanda Brewster, now at the Yale Global Health Leadership Institute. Others whose conversations helped shape ideas during this project include Professors Diana Eck, Richard Cash, P. Gregg Greenough, Satchit Balsari, Jennifer Leaning (again), and the design students of Professor Rahul Mehrotra, as well as Kalpesh Bhatt, Jenny Bordo, Deonnie Moodie, Leila Shayegan, and staff at the Harvard Global Health Institute. The Treese family keeps my longtime interest in India alive and relevant. An early version of Chapter 2 was delivered as a public lecture in the Duke University Keenan Institute for Ethics series at Duke Divinity School in April 2013. I thank Duke Professors Luke Bretherton and Ebrahim Moosa for the invitation, Dr. Raymond Barfield for his contagious enthusiasm about the health-faith connection, and Maria Doerfler for taking time out of a crushing week to be present. Abundant thanks also to the Duke students who asked hard questions and prodded me to take a stand on my politics, a rare (even strangely foreign) request for this early church historian trained in clinical science. I hope they might find here the kernels of more substantial responses to questions that were left hanging that evening.

The decision to include Henry Trevitt's public health journey in this book was complex from the start. At first the details seemed too personal and I imagined it for a different sort of story. But throughout work on this book, Henry's adventures kept poking in at the edges. It seemed fair to give him a whole chapter, if only as a cautionary lesson in the power of nineteenth-century politics and their pervasive influence on contemporary health policy. I thank Holly Cobb and others in my extended family for their presence during the long and often startling research on Henry. Thanks also to Matthew L. Lena, who first pointed me to several of the public records that helped fill the substantial documentary gap caused by Henry's various disasters. The library staff in the Special Collections archive at Princeton Theological Seminary in 2009 made it possible to consult the David and Jane Wales Trumbull Manuscript Collection pertaining to the Trevitts' tenure in Chile. A late draft of this chapter was much improved by the kind and generous rigor of Megan Marshall, who read it on short notice in an impossible time.

Cynthia Read and her editorial staff at Oxford University Press have now seen me through three books with uncommon sense, cheer, and professionalism. The book would not exist without their creative vision for what is possible, and the two anonymous external readers who promptly and warmly encouraged what was at first little more than a nascent and flickering idea.

I dedicate the book to the memory of a fellow writer, long-time friend, and spiritual mentor, Virginia Holland Andrews. From the moment we first met over drinks in a painter's studio in 1983 until her brave death to cancer in 2011, Gini was always ready to talk about ways to "push the envelope" on religion and writing. My life has been profoundly shaped by her model of grace and wisdom, an incarnation of hospitality into the healing space of a faith-filled crossing.

IMAGE CREDITS

Chapter 1 (facing page 1)
Benjamin Rush, Medical Inquiries and Observations, Second Edition (1789), here opened to page with "S. Saltmarsh" inscribed at top right. Author photo.

Chapter 2 (facing page 25)
Public Water Faucet. Author photo.

Chapter 3 (facing page 45)
Dr. Henry Trevitt's medical microscope (ca. 1850), shown here with his wife's rosary. Author photo.

Chapter 4 (facing page 83)
Eleanor Roosevelt and the United Nations Universal Declaration of Human Rights. US National Archives. Public domain.

Chapter 5 (facing page 125)
Religious health assets workshop participants in Zambia mapping the local religious health assets in their community. Photo courtesy of the African Religious Health Assets Programme. Used with permission.

Chapter 6 (facing page 163)
"Prosphoron" (gift) bread used in Orthodox Christian liturgy, seen here on the altar. The square central section used to celebrate the eucharist in the liturgy has been removed. This remaining loaf will be cut into small pieces and freely available to everyone present, regardless of religious identity. Photo by Jim Forest. Used with permission.

NOTES

Chapter 1

1. Alyn Brodsky, *Benjamin Rush: Patriot and Physician* (New York: St. Martin's Press, 2004), 5–6.
2. Brodsky, *Benjamin Rush*, 345.
3. Brodsky, *Benjamin Rush*, 346.
4. As quoted in "Benjamin Rush," *Dictionary of Unitarian and Universalist Biography*, http://uudb.org/articles/benjaminrush.html, accessed 12/26/13.
5. Brodsky, *Benjamin Rush*, 290.
6. He is listed as "Seth Saltmarsh, MD, 1837" in W. J. Maxwell, compiler, under direction of the Alumni Association of the University, *General Alumni Catalogue of the University of Pennsylvania* (Philadelphia: Alumni Association of the University, 1922), 505.
7. "William Trevitt," entry in *Biographical Encyclopedia of Ohio of the Nineteenth Century* (Cincinnati and Philadelphia: Galaxy Publishing Co., 1876), 158.
8. The one-volume second edition I have cited here is Benjamin Rush, *Medical Inquiries and Observations. To Which is Added an Appendix, Containing Observations on the Duties of a*

Physician and the Methods of Improving Medicine (Philadelphia and London, 1789), 254. As noted, the book was to go through a number of different editions and expansions, with different publishers and slight changes in the title and number of volumes before Rush's death in 1813; it seems to have settled into four volumes by 1809. As this quote suggests, Rush was a dedicated student of the works of Herman Boerhaave (1668–1738), a profoundly religious Dutch botanist, humanist, and physician who taught at the University of Leiden. Boerhaave is sometimes regarded as the founder of clinical medicine, that is, teaching medical students by direct clinical "bedside" experience.

9. William Staughton, *An Eulogium in Memory of the Late Dr. Benjamin Rush*, address delivered July 8, 1813, at the Second Presbyterian Church, Philadelphia, 31, https://archive.org/details/eulogiuminmemory00stau, accessed 2/21/14.

10. Benjamin Rush, *The Autobiography of Benjamin Rush: His "Travels Through Life" together with his Commonplace Book for 1789–1813*, ed. George W. Corner (Princeton, NJ: American Philosophical Society, 1948), 85, cited in Brodsky, *Benjamin Rush*, 254.

11. David Hosack, "Biographical Account of Dr. Benjamin Rush, of Philadelphia," *Annals of Philosophy* 8 (August 1816): 87.

12. Terms like "third world" or "developing/developed nations" are generally avoided today as being inaccurate as well as patronizing or belittling to the citizens and governments of such countries. It is now more common to refer to nations around the world—rich or poor—in terms of their World Bank economic classification, as "low-income countries" (LICs), "middle-income countries" (MICs), and "high-income countries" (HICs). Such classifications, however, are admittedly just another relative label externally imposed by a global organization of power and based on solely fiscal values. These terms also tend to gloss over the wide variations in power dynamics from wealth to poverty that are found within virtually every nation regardless of how its economics might be compared to other nations.

13. Jennifer Leaning, MD, SMH, lecture to Harvard undergraduates at a training session of the Harvard Global Health Institute's "Young Leaders for Global Health" program, February 20, 2013.

14. On the figure of 40 percent, see Katherine Marshall, "A Discussion with Reverend Canon Ted Karpf," Berkley Center for Religion, Peace & World Affairs, Georgetown University, November 13, 2010, http://berkleycenter.georgetown.edu/inte rviews/a-discussion-with-reverend-canon-ted-karpf, accessed 4/12/14.

15. On these diversities, see especially now Katherine Marshall, *Global Institutions of Religion: Ancient Movers, Modern Shakers*, Routledge Global Institutions Series (London: Routledge, 2013).

16. See, e.g., Melanie Tervalon and Jann Murray-García, "Cultural Humility versus Cultural Competence: A Critical Distinction in Defining Physician Training Outcomes in Multicultural Education," *Journal of Health Care for the Poor and Underserved* 9, no. 2 (1998): 117–25. Physician-anthropologist Dr. Paul Farmer's allusion to "cultural humility" is taken from a public dialogue with Harvard Divinity School Professor Davíd Carrasco on the occasion of the publication of *In the Company of the Poor: Conversations with Dr. Paul Farmer and Fr. Gustavo Gutiérrez*, ed. Michael Griffin and Jennie Weiss Bloch (Maryknoll, NY: Orbis Books, 2013). The event was sponsored by the Harvard Divinity School Science, Religion, and Culture Program and took place at First Church, Cambridge, Massachusetts, February 11, 2014.

17. Katherine Marshall, *Global Institutions of Religion*, 191.

18. Preamble to the Constitution of the World Health Organization 1946, as adopted by the International Health Conference, New York, June 19–July 22, 1946.

19. Charles Edward Amory Winslow, *The Evolution and Significance of the Modern Public Health Campaign* (New Haven: Yale University Press, 1923), quoted in Richard Skolnik, *Global Health 101*, 2nd ed. (Burlington, MA: Jones & Bartlett, 2012), 6.

20. Elizabeth Fee, "Public Health, Past and Present: A Shared Social Vision," in *A History of Public Health*, Expanded Edition, ed. George Rosen (Baltimore: Johns Hopkins University Press, 1993), xxxviii.

21. P. Gregg Greenough, Personal communication, 4/1/13. For the context, see "Public health at the world's largest gathering: A field report from India's Kumbh Mela," oral presentation, Harvard School of Public Health, March 28, 2013, http://webapps.sph.

harvard.edu/accordentG1/kumbhmela_20130328/index.htm, accessed 2/21/14.

22. "Social Determinants of Health: Key Concepts," World Health Organization, http://www.who.int/social_determinants/thecom mission/finalreport/key_concepts/en/, accessed 5/2/14.

23. On the 1978 Alma Ata Declaration, see the World Health Organization, "Declaration of Alma Ata: International Conference on Primary Health Care, Alma Ata, USSR, 6–12 September 1978," http://www.who.int/publications/almaata_ declaration_en.pdf, accessed 8/16/14. For discussion, see, e.g., Matthew Basilico, Jonathan Weigel, Anjali Motgi, Jacob Bor, and Salmaan Keshavjee, "Health for All? Competing Theories and Geopolitics," in *Reimagining Global Health: An Introduction*, ed. Paul Farmer, Jim Yong Kim, Arthur Kleinman, and Matthew Basilico (Berkeley: University of California Press, 2013), 74–110. For an excerpt from Virchow's classic report, see Rudolf Carl Virchow, "Report on the Typhus Epidemic in Upper Silesia" [Voices from the Past], *American Journal of Public Health* 96, no. 12 (2006): 2102–05. For the original, see Rudolf Carl Virchow, *Archiv für pathologische Anatomie und Physiologie und für klinische Medicin*, Vol. 2 (Berlin: George Reimer, 1848), 143–332. For an English translation of the entire report, see Rudolf Carl Virchow, *Collected Essays on Public Health and Epidemiology*, Vol. 1, ed. L. J. Rather (Boston: Science History Publications, 1985), 204–319.

24. As quoted in Vicente Navarro, "What We Mean by Social Determinants of Health," *International Journal of Health Services* 39, no. 3 (2009): 441.

25. Orielle Solar and Alec Irwin, *A Conceptual Framework for Action on the Social Determinants of Health*, Social Determinants of Health Discussion Paper 2 (Policy and Practice) (Geneva: World Health Organization, 2010), 11, http://www.who.int/sdhconference/resources/Conceptual-frameworkforactiononSDH_eng.pdf, accessed 5/2/14.

26. Commission on Social Determinants of Health, *Closing the Gap in a Generation: Health Equity Through Action on the Social Determinants of Health Commission on Social Determinants*

of Health Final Report (Geneva: World Health Organization, 2008). See also, Michael Marmot and Richard G. Wilkinson, eds., *Social Determinants of Health*, 2nd ed., (New York: Oxford University Press, 2005); Vicente Navarro, "What we mean by Social Determinants of Health," 423–41; and Michael Marmot, Jessica Allen, Ruth Bell, Ellen Bloomer, and Peter Goldblatt on behalf of the Consortium for the European Review of Social Determinants of Health and the Health Divide, "WHO European Review of Social Determinants of Health and the Health Divide," *The Lancet* 380 (September 15, 2012): 1011–29, http://dx.doi.org/10.1016/S0140-6736(12)61228-8, accessed 5/2/14.

27. In discussion about the most appropriate subtitle for this book, for example, I informally surveyed twenty individuals whose work was evenly distributed between religion and health, to ask which phrase would draw their interest more: public health, global health, or world health. Of the eighteen who responded, sixteen instantly preferred global health. Only one person (who had no health science background) preferred "public health." And while the lone individual who preferred "world health" suggested it as a way to avoid the emerging stereotype now associated with the discipline of "global health," another respondent was equally insistent that "world health" should not be used because it was an unknown term that would have little meaning for the reader.

28. Anne Sebert Kuhlmann and Lora Iannotti, "Resurrecting 'International' and 'Public' in Global Health: Has the Pendulum Swung Too Far?" *American Journal of Public Health* 104, no. 4 (2014): 585.

29. For my view on and understanding of the phrase "global health," I have been most influenced by the global health framework and understanding of Dr. Sue J. Goldie, founding faculty director of the Harvard Global Health Institute. While deeply informed by Dr. Goldie's inspiration and vision, my description and explanations in this chapter do not necessarily reflect her views and should not be taken as representative of her multidimensional and deeply nuanced understanding of this concept. My intention here is, rather,

to reflect principally a perception of global health's definition as it relates to the potential for a faith-based lens, the focus of this book.

30. On this and related ideas, see Anne-Emanuelle Birn, "The politics of global health agenda-setting," The 2012 Stephen Stewart Gloyd Endowed Lecture, University of Washington School of Public Health, October 5, 2012, http://www.youtube.com/watch?v=HQ3cv9-CaVI, accessed 12/27/13.

31. Anne-Emanuelle Birn, Yogan Pillay, and Timothy H. Holtz, eds., *Textbook of International Health: Global Health in a Dynamic World*, 3rd ed. (New York: Oxford University Press, 2009), 6. For further discussion about global health and its practice and potential, see, e.g., Richard Skolnik, *Global Health 101*.

32. *The Lancet*—University of Oslo Commission on Global Governance for Health, "The Political Origins of Health Inequity: Prospects for Change," *The Lancet* 383, no. 9917 (2014): 661. For a recent book that explores some of the creative areas where a multidisciplinary approach to global health draws on a variety of religious ideas and global practices, see Ellen L. Idler, ed., *Religion as a Social Determinant of Public Health: Interdisciplinary Inquiries* (New York: Oxford University Press, 2014).

33. *Shorter Oxford English Dictionary*, 6th Edition (New York: Oxford University Press, 2007), vol. 1, p. 214.

34. Marjorie Anderson and Blanche Colton Williams, *Old English Handbook* (Boston: Houghton Mifflin, 1935), 378.

35. Ted A. Campbell, *John Wesley and Christian Antiquity: Religious Vision and Cultural Change* (Nashville, TN: Kingswood Books, 1991), 1.

Chapter 2

1. On the every-twelve-year Kumbh Mela in Allahabad, India, the most comprehensive historical source is Kama Maclean, *Pilgrimage and Power: The Kumbh Mela in Allahabad, 1765–1954* (New York: Oxford University Press, 2008). For more information about the Harvard University 2013 Kumbh Mela research project, see http://southasiainstitute.harvard.edu/

kumbh-mela/, accessed 2/25/14. See also Tom Downey, "What Urban Planners Can Learn from a Hindu Religious Festival," *Smithsonian Magazine,* September 2013, http://www.smithsonianmag.com/travel/what-urban-planners-can-le arn-from-a-hindu-religious-festival-903131/, accessed 2/25/14. For the 2013 estimate of one hundred million pilgrims, see, e.g., Mark Memmott, " 'Biggest gathering on earth' begins in India; Kumbh Mela may draw 100 million," *NPR* January 14, 2013, http://www.npr.org/blogs/thetwo-way/2013/01/14/169313222/ biggest-gathering-on-earth-begins-in-india-kumbh-mela-ma y-draw-100-million, accessed 9/15/13. For the estimate of thirty million on February 10, see Soutik Biswas, "India's Kumbh Mela Festival Holds Most Auspicious Day," *BBC News India,* February 10, 2013, http://www.bbc.co.uk/news/ world-asia-india-21395425, accessed 9/15/13. I thank Kalpesh Bhatt for sharing with me his experience during the 2001 Gujarat earthquake; it should be noted that the text I give as dialogue in this chapter is a paraphrase based on my rough notes (later shared with Kalpesh) which were recorded from memory immediately following that Sunday lunch conversation.

2. Steve de Gruchy, Nico Koopman, and Sytse Strijbos, eds., *From Our Side: Emerging Perspectives on Development and Ethics* (Amsterdam: Rozenberg Publishers/West Lafayette, IN: Purdue University Press, 2008), 281.

3. Francis X. Clooney, SJ, *Comparative Theology: Deep Learning Across Religious Borders* (Malden, MA: Wiley-Blackwell, 2010), 15–16.

4. Clooney, *Comparative Theology,* 15–16.

5. Clooney, *Comparative Theology,* 165.

6. On pilgrimage as border crossing, see Victor and Edith Turner, *Image and Pilgrimage in Christian Culture,* originally published in 1978, reprinted with a new introduction by Deborah Ross, Columbia Classics in Religion (New York: Columbia University Press, 2011).

7. Robert Doran, trans., *The Lives of Simeon Stylites,* Cistercian Studies Series 112 (Kalamazoo, MI: Cistercian Publications, 1992), 82–83 (on his arbitration) and 159 (on interest rates).

8. Susan Ashbrook Harvey, "Foreword," In Doran, *The Lives of Simeon Stylites*, 11.

9. *Si-Yu-Ki: Buddhist Records of the Western World, Translated from the Chinese of Hiuen Tsiang (AD 629)*, trans. Samuel Beal (London: Trübner and Co, 1884; reprinted Delhi: Oriental Books Reprint Corp., 1969); the account of his visit to Prayag (the ancient name for modern Allahabad, also known as Prayaga) and the story of the festival and rich prince's divestment is in Book 5, 230–34. The account of Huien Tsang is also found in Thomas Watters, Thomas William Rhys Davids, Stephen Wootton Bushell, and Vincent Arthur Smith, *On Yuan Chwang's Travels in India, 629–645 AD*, Oriental Translation Fund New Series 14 (London: Royal Asiatic Society, 1904), esp. 363–65. As these sources suggest, his name has many variant spellings, including also Xuanzang and Hsüan Tsang.

10. Diana Eck, *Darśan: Seeing the Divine Image in India*, 3rd ed. (New York: Columbia University Press, 1998), 3.

11. See, e.g., David Morgan, *The Sacred Gaze: Religious Visual Culture in Theory and Practice* (Berkeley: University of California Press, 2005); Georgia Frank, *The Memory of the Eyes: Pilgrims to Living Saints in Christian Late Antiquity*, Transformation of the Classical Heritage 30 (Berkeley: University of California Press, 2000); and Patricia Cox Miller, *The Corporeal Imagination: Signifying the Holy in Late Ancient Christianity*, Divinations: Rereading Late Ancient Religion (Philadelphia: University of Pennsylvania Press, 2009).

12. *The Travels of Fa-hsien (399–414 A.D.), or Record of the Buddhistic Kingdoms*, trans. H. A. Giles (New York: Cambridge University Press, 1923, repr. 2011), 48.

13. Diana Eck, personal communication, November 2012.

14. For the claim that the 1817 Kumbh Mela triggered the worldwide nineteenth-century global cholera pandemic, see Ziad A. Memish, Gwen M. Stephens, Robert Steffen, and Qanta A. Ahmed, "Emergence of Medicine for Mass Gatherings: Lessons from the Hajj," *The Lancet Infectious Diseases* 12, no.1 (2012): 56–65, at 57. Memish and colleagues draw on J. N. Hays, *Epidemics and Pandemics: Their Impacts on Human History*

(Santa Barbara, California: ABC-CLIO, 2005), esp. 193–200 and 217 for this claim. On the history of cholera at the Kumbh Mela itself over the past two hundred years (at Allahabad and several other cities in India where the festival takes place in interim years), see, e.g., A. Leslie Banks, "Religious Fairs and Festivals in India," *The Lancet* 277, no. 7169 (January 21, 1961), 162–63; S. C. Bagchi and S. C. Banerjee, "The Kumbh Fair (1966): Aspects of Environmental Sanitation and Other Related Measures," *Indian Journal of Public Health* 11, no. 4 (1967): 180–84; A. D. M. Bryceson., "Cholera, the Flickering Flame," *Proceedings of the Royal Society of Medicine* 70 (1977): 363–65; "Sanitary Reform in India: IV. Sanitary Reports," *The Lancet* 171, no. 4411 (March 21, 1908): 883–84; and more generally, H. Herbert, "The Natural History of Hardwar Fair Cholera Outbreaks," *The Lancet* 146, no. 3752 (July 27, 1895): 201–02.

15. On St. Julitta, see Basil of Caesarea, "On the Martyr Julitta," trans. Susan R. Holman, in *St. Basil the Great on Fasting and Feasts*, trans. Susan R. Holman and Mark DelCogliano, Popular Patristics Series 50 (Yonkers, NY: St. Vladimir Seminary Press, 2013), 16–21 and 109–22.

16. The reference to Basil's hospital being just outside the city walls of Caesarea is in Gregory of Nazianzus, *Oration* 44.63.

17. Now a museum, it is considered "one of the pre-eminent monuments of Seljuk architecture." For an overview and images, see http://gevhernesibe.erciyes.edu.tr, accessed 1/15/12.

18. See, e.g., Robert Doran, trans., *Stewards of the Poor: The Man of God, Rabbula, and Hiba in Fifth-Century Edessa*, Cistercian Studies Series 208 (Kalamazoo, MI: Cistercian Publications, 2006).

19. See, e.g., "The Life of our Holy Father, John the Almsgiver," in *Three Byzantine Saints*, ed. and trans. Elizabeth Dawes and Norman H. Baynes (Crestwood, NY: St. Vladimir's Seminary Press, 1977), 195–270.

20. For more on hospitals in the Middle East in late antiquity, see, e.g., Andrew T. Crislip, *From Monastery to Hospital: Christian Monasticism and the Transformation of Health Care in Late Antiquity* (Grand Rapids: University of Michigan Press, 2005);

Andrew T. Crislip, *Thorns in the Flesh: Illness and Sanctity in Late Ancient Christianity*, Divinations: Rereading Late Ancient Religion (Philadelphia: University of Pennsylvania Press, 2013); and Guenter B. Risse, *Mending Bodies, Saving Souls: A History of Hospitals* (New York: Oxford University Press, 1999). For William Trevitt on mineral springs in Ohio in the nineteenth century, see William Trevitt, W. W. Dawson, Theo. G. Wormley, and John G. F. Holston, "Dr. Trevitt, From the Committee on the Mineral Waters of Ohio," *The Ohio Medical and Surgical Journal* 9, no. 4 (1857): 283–96.

21. Joseph Lumbard, "Some Reflections on Hospitality in Islam," in *Hosting the Stranger: Between Religions*, ed. Richard Kearney and James Taylor (New York: Continuum, 2011), 133.

22. Institute of Medicine of the National Academies of Science, Food and Nutrition Board, Standing Committee on the Scientific Evaluation of Dietary Reference Intakes, *Dietary Reference Intakes for Water, Potassium, Sodium, Chloride, and Sulfate* (Washington, DC: The National Academies Press, 2005), http://www.nal.usda.gov/fnic/DRI//DRI_Water/water_full_report. pdf, accessed 1/21/14. Originally known as the Recommended Dietary Allowances (RDAs), this national nutrition standard was established in 1941 and broadened and renamed Dietary Reference Intake in 1997.

23. For more information about these rights, see, e.g., Office of the United Nations High Commission for Human Rights, UN Habitat, and World Health Organization, *The Right to Water: Fact Sheet 35* (Geneva: OHCHR, 2010), http://www.ohchr.org/Documents/Publications/FactSheet35en.pdf, accessed 1/21/14; and Jean Ziegler, Christophe Golay, Claire Mahon, Sally-Anne Way, *The Fight for the Right to Food: Lessons Learned* (Geneva: Palgrave Macmillan, 2011). For recent examples of the effect of disregarding the human need for food and water at a national level as it relates to international public policies in Haiti, see, e.g., Center for Human Rights and Global Justice (CHRGJ), RFK Center for Justice and Human Rights, Partners In Health, and Zanmi Lasante, *Wòch Nan Soley: The Denial of the Right to Water in Haiti* (June 2008), http://parthealth.3cdn.

net/0badc680352663967e_v6m6b1ayx.pdf, accessed 1/21/14; and Center for Human Rights and Global Justice (CHRGJ), RFK Center for Justice and Human Rights, Partners In Health, and Zanmi Lasante, *Sak Vid Pa Kanpe: The Impact of US Food Aid on Human Rights in Haiti* (2010), http://parthealth.3cdn. net/3f82f61a3316d7f1a0_pvm6b80f3.pdf, accessed 1/21/14.

24. United Nations General Assembly, resolution A/64/292, adopted September 24, 2010. A resolution is not a law; for the legal nuances of water rights, see, e.g., Sharmila L. Murthy, "The Human Right(s) to Water and Sanitation: History, Meaning and the Controversy Over Privatization," *Berkeley Journal of International Law* 31, no. 1 (2013), 89-149.

25. Gerrit Bos, trans., *Qusṭā ibn Lūqā al-Baʿlabakkī's Medical Regime for the Pilgrims to Mecca: The Risāla fī tadbīr safar al-hajj,* Islamic Philosophy, Theology and Science: Texts and Studies 11 (Leiden: E. J. Brill, 1992), 57; for water (chapters 8-10), see 57-64.

26. Bos, *Qusṭā ibn Lūqā al-Baʿlabakkī's Medical Regime for the Pilgrims to Mecca,* 59.

27. Bos, *Qusṭā ibn Lūqā al-Baʿlabakkī's Medical Regime for the Pilgrims to Mecca,* 17.

28. On Christian doctors in Mecca, see Bos, *Qusṭā ibn Lūqā al-Baʿlabakkī's Medical Regime for the Pilgrims to Mecca* 85, n. 5. On William Wey's advice about water, see Francis Davey, ed. and trans., *The Itineraries of William Wey* (Oxford: The Bodleian Library, 2010), 27. Another pilgrimage text not discussed here but intriguing for its inclusion as part of a medical manuscript is that of Wey's contemporary, Richard of Lincoln, whose Middle English "Pilgrimage to Jerusalem" is a verbal mapping of place, distance, and salvific relics for veneration along the way, contained within an English medical and astrological compendium dated to 1454 (Wellcome Library MS 8004). The pilgrimage account by itself (ff. 75-84v) is now available in an edited translation; see Francis Davey, *Richard of Lincoln: A Medieval Doctor Travels to Jerusalem* (Exeter, UK: Azure Publications, 2013). I am grateful to the Daveys and to publishers Robin and Diane Wilks for their phenomenally kind and rapid response in sending me a copy of this new translation.

29. Tracy L. Prowse, Henry P. Schwarcz, Shelley R. Saunders, Roberto Macchiarelli, and Luca Bondioli, "Isotopic Evidence for Age-Related Variation in Diet from Isola Sacra, Italy," *American Journal of Physical Anthropology* 128 (2005): 2–13. Isotopes, for example from dental samples, can reveal whether a population was local or represented persons who had migrated to the area at some point during their lifetime. See, e.g., T. L. Prowse, H. P. Schwarcz, P. Garnsey, M. Knyf, R. Macchiarelli, and L. Bondioli, "Isotopic Evidence for Age-Related Immigration to Imperial Rome," *American Journal of Physical Anthropology* 132 (2007): 510–19.

30. Tracy L. Prowse, "Bioarchaeological Investigation of Life and Death on a Roman Imperial Estate," lecture presented at "How Bodies Matter: The Intersection of Science, Religion, and the Humanities in the Study of the Ancient Mediterranean World," Harvard Divinity School, Cambridge, Mass., March 15–16, 2013.

31. T. L. Prowse, S. R. Saundiers, H. P. Schwarcz, P. Garnsey, R. Macchiarelli, and L. Bondioli, "Isotopic and Dental Evidence for Infant and Young Child Feeding Practices in an Imperial Roman Skeletal Sample," *American Journal of Physical Anthropology* 137 (2008): 294–308. See also Tracy L. Prowse, "Diet and Dental Health Through the Life Course in Roman Italy," in *Social Bioarchaeology*, ed. Sabrina C. Agarwal and Bonnie A. Glencross (Malden, MA: Wiley-Blackwell, 2011), 410–37.

32. Luigi Capasso, "Indoor Pollution and Respiratory Diseases in Ancient Rome" [letter], *The Lancet* 356 (2000): 1774. See also L. Capasso, [Archaeological Documentation of the Atmospheric Pollution in Antiquity](article in Italian), *Med. Secoli* 7, no. 3 (1995): 35–44; For abstract in English, see Pubmed Abstract PMID 11623479.

33. Luigi Capasso and Luisa Di Domenicantonio, "Work-related Syndesmoses on the Bones of Children Who Died at Herculaneum," [Letter] *The Lancet* 352, no. 9140 (1998): 1634.

34. Ibid.

35. Leonard V. Rutgers, "Catacombs and Health," in *Children and Family in Late Antiquity: Life, Death and Interaction*, ed. Christian Laes, Katariina Mustakallio, and Ville Vuolanto

(Leuven: Peeters, in press); see also, L.V. Rutgers, M. van Strydonck, M. Boudin, and C. van der Linde, "Stable Isotope Data from the Early Christian Catacombs of Ancient Rome: New Insights into the Dietary Habits of Rome's Early Christians," *Journal of Archaeological Science* 36 (2009): 1127–34.

36. See, e.g., Kyle Harper, *Slavery in the Late Roman World AD 275–425* (New York: Cambridge University Press, 2011).

37. See, e.g., Susan Guise Sheridan, "New Life the Dead Receive: The Relationship between Human Remains and the Cultural Record for Byzantine St. Stephen's," *Revue Biblique* 106, no. 4 (1999): 574–611.

38. Barry Kemp, Anna Stevens, Gretchen R. Dabbs, Melissa Zabecki, and Jerome C. Rose, "Life, Death and Beyond in Akhenaton's Egypt: Excavating the South Tombs Cemetery at Amarna," *Antiquity* 87 (2013): 64–78; for a general study of the dig, see Barry Kemp, *The City of Akhenaten and Nefertiti: Amarna and its People*, New Aspects of Antiquity (London: Thames and Hudson, 2014).

39. A. Bagus Laksana, "Comparative Theology: Between Identity and Alterity," in *The New Comparative Theology: Interreligious Insights from the Next Generation*, ed. Francis X. Clooney (London: T&T Clark, 2010), 19.

40. "shaped . . . by its culture." For this phrase and an introduction into the bone research summarized in this chapter, I am indebted to Steven Friesen and Laura Nasrallah, co-directors of the research colloquium "How Bodies Matter: The Intersection of Science, Religion, and the Humanities in the Study of the Ancient Mediterranean World," Harvard Divinity School, March 15–16, 2013.

Chapter 3

1. John Trevitt to Henry Trevitt, May 16, 1846, unpublished letter, collection of the author.

2. Sarah Jane Trevitt's narrative genealogy was published, with minor variants (and a few errors), in Charles James Smith, *History of the Town of Mont Vernon, New Hampshire*

(Boston: Blanchard Printing Co., 1907), "Genealogy," 157–58. Smith's book also contains Sarah Jane's drawing of the old Mont Vernon Meeting House (following p. 84, cited on Smith, p. iv). In this chapter I have relied most on the narrative as it is found in an unpublished transcript of the original in Ellen Trevitt's handwriting and preserved in family archives.

3. *The Biographical Encyclopedia of Ohio of the Nineteenth Century* (Cincinnati and Philadelphia: Galaxy Publishing Co., 1876), 157, http://quod.lib.umich.edu/m/moa/AHU5132.0001. 001?view=toc, accessed 5/23/14. On the older Dr. John Trevitt's appointment and his death in Augusta, Georgia, on August 18, 1821, see also Charles Kitchell Gardner, *Dictionary of All Officers Who Have Been Commissioned or Have Been Appointed and Served in the Army of the United States, Since the Inauguration of Their First President in 1789, to the First January 1853* (New York: G. P. Putnam and Company, 1853), 453.

4. *The Biographical Encyclopedia of Ohio of the Nineteenth Century*, 158, http://quod.lib.umich.edu/m/moa/AHU5132.0001. 001? view=toc, accessed 5/23/14.

5. Michael B. Katz, *In the Shadow of the Poorhouse: A Social History of Welfare in America* (New York: Basic Books, 1986), 291.

6. The literature on the nineteenth-century public welfare system in America is extensive. For representative sources, see, e.g., F. B. Sanborn, *The Public Charities of Massachusetts during the Century ending Jan. 1, 1876: Report made to the Massachusetts Centennial Commission, Feb. 1, 1876, under Direction of the Massachusetts Board of State Charities* (Boston: Wright and Potter State Printers, 1876); and David Wagner, *The Poorhouse: America's Forgotten Institution* (Lanham, MD: Rowan and Littlefield, 2005); See also Charles E. Rosenberg, *The Care of Strangers: The Rise of America's Hospital System* (New York: Basic Books, 1987). On the relationship between the history of American public health as it relates to health issues caused by political displacement and international refugees, I have been especially inspired by Kathryn Hulme, *The Wild Place* (Boston: Little Brown, 1953), and S. Josephine Baker, *Fighting*

for Life (New York: Macmillan Publishing Co., 1939, reprinted: Huntington, NY: Robert E. Krieger Publishing Co. Inc., 1980).

7. Alyn Brodsky, *Benjamin Rush: Patriot and Physician* (New York: St. Martin's Press, 2004), 105.

8. Ezra Stiles Ely, *A Sermon for the Rich to Buy that they may Benefit Themselves and the Poor* (New York: Williams and Whiting, 1810), 19–20.

9. See, e.g., Columbus, Ohio 1856 map, http://www.ohiomemory. org/cdm/compoundobject/collection/p267401coll32/id/16715/ show/16709/rec/134, accessed 2/21/14.

10. See, e.g., Demetrios Constantelos, *Byzantine Philanthropy and Social Welfare* (New Brunswick, NJ: Rutgers University Press, 1968); Timothy S. Miller, *The Birth of the Hospital in the Byzantine Empire* (Baltimore: Johns Hopkins Press, 1997); Andrew Crislip, *From Monastery to Hospital: Christian Monasticism and the Transformation of Health Care in Antiquity* (Grand Rapids: University of Michigan Press, 2005); and idem, *Thorns in the Flesh: Illness and Sanctity in Late Antique Christianity* (Philadelphia: University of Pennsylvania Press, 2012).

11. Perhaps the best-known story is that of the prostitutes, "rescued" by the empress Theodora in sixth-century Constantinople, who, Procopius says, threw themselves from the high windows of their prison rather than suffer such enforced "reform." Procopius, *Secret History*, trans. Richard Atwater (Ann Arbor: University of Michigan Press, 1963), 84. The late fourth-century bishop, Firmus of Caesarea, also describes how some of those whose care was funded by housing them in the local poorhouse ran away; Firmus of Caesarea, *Ep.* 43, in Marie-Ange Calvet-Sebasti and Pierre-Louis Gatier, ed. and trans., *Firmus de Césarée: Lettres*, Sources Chrétiennes 350 (Paris: Les Éditions du Cerf, 1989), n.p.

12. See, e.g., Lee Palmer Wandel, *Always Among Us: Images of the Poor in Zwingli's Zurich* (New York: Cambridge University Press, 1990); Carter Lindberg, *Beyond Charity: Reformation Initiatives for the Poor* (Minneapolis: Fortress Press, 1993); and André Biéler, *Calvin's Economic and Social Thought*, trans. James Grieg (Geneva: World Alliance of Reformed Churches/

World Council of Churches, 2005). I thank Frank Sadowski for introducing me to Biéler's work.

13. Ely, *A Sermon for the Rich*.

14. Ely, *A Sermon for the Rich*, 24. For more on Ely's work, see Rosenberg, *The Care of Strangers*, 15–18. For Ely's detailed account of the poorhouse, see Ezra Stiles Ely, *The Second Journal of the Stated Preacher to the Hospital and Almshouse in the City of New York for a Part of the Year of Our Lord 1813* (Philadelphia: M. Cary, 1815).

15. James Priestley, *A Charity Sermon Delivered in the Methodist Chapel, Halifax (Nova Scotia) on the Evening of Christmas Day* (Halifax: A. H. Holland, 1818).

16. Priestley, *A Charity Sermon*, 11.

17. Priestley, *A Charity Sermon*, 12.

18. For the full text and translation, see "The Shepherd of Hermas," trans. Bart D. Ehrman, *The Apostolic Fathers*, Loeb Classical Library 25, 2 vols. (Cambridge, MA: Harvard University Press, 2003), 2:162–473; the parable of the elm and the vine (Book 3, Similitude 2) is at 308–15. For further discussion of this parable, see Carolyn Osiek, *Rich and Poor in the Shepherd of Hermas: An Exegetical-Social Investigation*, The Catholic Biblical Quarterly Monograph Series 15 (Washington, DC: The Catholic Biblical Association of America, 1983).

19. John Stanford, *An Address Delivered in the Orphan Asylum, New York, February 5, 1822, on the Conflagration of the Orphan House in the City of Philadelphia on the 23rd of January* (New York: E. Conrad, 1822).

20. Stanford, *An Address Delivered in the Orphan Asylum*, n.p.

21. Samuel Hayes Elliott, *New England's Chattels: or, Life in the Northern Poor House* (New York: H. Dayton, 1858).

22. Matthew Carey, *Essays on the Public Charities of Philadelphia, Intended to Vindicate the Benevolent Societies of this City from the Charge of Encouraging Idleness, and to Place in Strong Relief, before an Enlightened Public, the Sufferings and Oppression under which the Greater Part of the Females Labour, Who Depend on Their Industry for a Support for Themselves and Children*, 4th ed. (Philadelphia: J. Clarke, 1829).

23. Dorothea L. Dix, *Remarks on Prisons and Prison Discipline in the United States* (Boston: Munroe & Francis, 1845), 45 (on ventilation), 56 (on moral deficiency).

24. James Bradley Finley, *Memorials of Prison Life*, ed. Rev. B. F. Tefft (Cincinnati: L. Swormstedt & A. Poe, 1853); see also Charles Chester Cole Jr., *Lion of the Forest: James B. Finley, Frontier Reformer* (Lexington, KY: University Press of Kentucky, 1994).

25. Finley, *Memorials of Prison Life*, 220.

26. James Grant Wilson and John Fiske, *Appleton's Cyclopaedia of American Biography* (New York: Appleton, 1892), vol. 3, p. 243, as cited in Amy E. Cummings, "Mary Jane Holmes and the Triumph of Fashion in *Ethelyn's Mistake*," in *Styling Texts: Dressing and Fashion in Literature*, ed. Cynthia G. Kuhn and Cindy L. Carlson (Youngstown, NY: Cambria Press, 2007), 150.

27. For her description of life in the nineteenth-century poorhouse, see, e.g., Mary J. Holmes, *English Orphans* (New York: J. H. Sears, 1855).

28. Margarette Daniels, "David Trumbull," in idem, *Makers of South America* (New York: Missionary Education Movement of the US and Canada, 1916), 188.

29. Daniels, "David Trumbull," 190.

30. Daniels, "David Trumbull," 191–92.

31. Daniels, "David Trumbull," 194.

32. Michelle Prain B., "La Iglesia Saint Paul's de Valparaíso, Patrimonio Tangible e intangible de la era Victoriana," *Revista Archivum* 5, no. 6 (2006): 174–92.

33. Irven Paul, *A Yankee Reformer in Chile: The Life and Works of David Trumbull* (South Pasadena, CA: William Carey Library, 1973). See also H. McKennie Goodpasture, "David Trumbull: Missionary Journalist and Liberty in Chile, 1845–1889," *Journal of Presbyterian History* 56, no. 2 (Summer 1978): 149–65. It is Goodpasture (157) who spells out Trumbull's affiliation as a Congregationalist serving the Presbyterian mission. See also Daniels, *Makers of South America*, 185–202. A train was available (though substantial discomforts remained) across the Panama isthmus by the late 1850s; the

Panama Canal would not be opened until 1914. For further details, see, e.g., John Haskell Kemble, *The Panama Route 1848–1869* (Columbus, SC: University of South Carolina Press, 1990).

34. "Dr. Trevitt has got an office," *Ohio State Journal* 47, no. 17 (July 22, 1857): 2. On the treasury fraud, see, e.g., "Wm. D. Morgan—The Newark Advocate—The Late Defalcation," *Ohio State Journal*, 47, no. 13 (June 24, 1857): 2.

35. These dates are taken from William Trevitt's three letters written during his sea voyage to his colleagues in Ohio and published in the *Ohio Medical and Surgical Journal* on May 1, 1858 (p. 378) and July 1, 1858 (p. 513).

36. William's active role in medical education and the ethics of medical training is documented in the Ohio State Medical Society minutes, published during the 1850s in the *Ohio Medical and Surgical Journal*; see, e.g., vol. 3, no. 6 (July 1, 1851), vol. 8, no. 6 (July 1, 1856), and vol. 9, no. 4 (March 1, 1857).

37. William Trevitt, "A Report on Asiatic Cholera Epidemic: To the Directors of the Ohio Penitentiary, Columbus, 30th November 1849," reprinted in *The Ohio State Medical Journal* 50 (September 1954): 860–62.

38. William Trevitt, "Dr. Trevitt's Letter on Cholera," in Joel Roberts, *The Cholera of 1849, and the Opinions of Medical and Other Professional Gentlemen, in Regards to its Origin and Proper Treatment, Embracing the Alopathy, Homoeopathy, Electrical and Eclectic Theories and Prescriptions, Selected from the Various Journals of the Day* (Sandusky City, Ohio: W. S. Mills and Co., 1850), 25. On William's reputation during the 1832 epidemic as a "skillful physician [who] saved every case he reached before the patient got into a certain condition," and who responded so fast that "[t]wo of his horses dropped dead under the spur," see Ephraim S. Colborn, *History of Fairfield and Perry Counties: Their Past and Present*, compiled by A. A. Graham (Chicago: W. H. Beers & Co., 1883), vol. 2, p. 310.

39. William Trevitt, W. W. Dawson, Theo G. Wormley and John G. F. Holston, "Report from the Committee on the Mineral Waters of Ohio," *The Ohio Medical and Surgical Journal* 9, no. 4 (March 1, 1857): 283–96.

40. The reference to William's initiative at smallpox inoculation is found in his annual report on prison medicine, titled "Ohio Penitentiary" and published in the *Daily Ohio Statesman*, 4, no. 34 (June 18, 1850): 1.

41. See above for William's three sea letters.

42. Wilhelm Trevitt Knappe, reminiscence on "Dr. William Trevitt," in Knappe's colorful late-in-life memoir, *History of the Wabash Valley*, n.d., 23–25; the reference to Lincoln is at p. 23, https://archive.org/details/historyofwabashv00knap, accessed 5/23/14.

43. "From Chile: Washington's Birthday at Valparaiso, the Indians['] Relations with the United States Varieties," *The New York Times*, April 11, 1860, briefly describes a report from Valparaiso's "City Hospital," an institution praised for having facilities such as a chapel, 255 beds, a dispensary, a room for bathing, and a laundry; during 1859 this City Hospital had provided care, the report says, to 3,207 patients. The description is a marked contrast to the author's view of the American Hospital, described further below.

44. Henry Trevitt's passport application, dated May 6, 1858, requests the passport "as soon as convenient as he [Henry] wishes to leave here as soon as it can be got." A. P. Russell, to Lewis Cass, May 6, 1858 (Washington, DC: United States Passport Office. National Archives and Records Administration, reel 70 [May 3–22, 1858]), document no. 7221, p. 385, https://archive.org/details/passportapplicat070unit, accessed 2/25/14. I thank Matthew L. Lena for first bringing this document to my attention.

45. "From Valparaiso: Shipping Intelligence—Insurrectionary Movements—General News," *The New York Times*, January 29, 1859, p. 1. While the *Times* attributes the boy's insanity to "intense study," the Washington, DC, correspondent of the Cleveland *National Democrat* reported to readers in William's home city of Columbus what is more likely the true story ("Dr. William Trevitt," *The Daily Ohio Statesman*, 5, no. 200, January 22, 1859: 2):

> A letter has been received . . . from a friend in Valparaiso, stating that by the recent destructive fire in that city,

Dr. Wm. Trevitt, U.S. Consul, and formerly Secretary of the State of Ohio, was a severe loser, his entire household furniture having been destroyed. In addition to this, the letter states that a son of the Doctor's was so affected by fright on the occasion, as to deprive him of his reason. This will indeed be sad news to Mr. Trevitt's numerous friends in your State.

46. Ellen M. Knights to Mr. I. E. Sanborn, March 31, 1850, http://www.maritimeheritage.org/PassLists/colorado49.html, accessed 12/16/13.
47. "Further about Dr. Trevitt and Ramirez, Full Account of the Affair," *Daily Ohio Statesman* 5, no. 286 (May 1, 1859): 2, notes the building as "situated among the hills, some half a mile from the city." While William Trevitt is mentioned frequently in the newspapers related to the consular crisis, I have found only two newspaper references that explicitly name Henry in Valparaiso between the fall of 1858 and 1860. One is his appointment replacing Dr. Thomas Page at the American Hospital; the other is Rand's account of March 27, 1859 (see below), and cited at length in this chapter. The villa is identified as belonging to the Venega family in "The Difficulty at Valparaiso," *Daily Ohio Statesman* 5, no. 283 (April 28, 1859): 2, in a section of that story attributed to "Correspondence of the *New York Times*."
48. All quotes in what follows from Charles Rand's account are from "Interesting from Valparaiso—Particulars of the attack on the Residence of Dr. Trevitt, the American Consul," *The Daily Ohio Statesman* 5, no. 294 (May 11, 1859): 2. The account of fleeing insurgents here is from *The New York Daily Tribune,* Thursday, March 31, 1859, p. 1, citing a report "From Our Own Correspondent," dated "Panama, March 22, 1859."
49. Rand's purported association with the Riobos is from "South American News," *San Francisco Bulletin* 8, no. 21 (May 2, 1859): Supplement p. 2. Lucinda Trevitt's obituary, nearly forty years later, includes an otherwise unattested detail about the fight, noting that "the doctor grappled with the captain, and in an attempt to secure the latter's sword four of his fingers

were almost completely severed from his hand. He secured the sword or rather cavalry saber, and it is yet in the possession of the family." While the obituary garbles many facts (e.g., dating the 1859 Valparaiso attack to 1868 in Peru), this particular detail about William's hand injury could be true, given that it was written by someone who would have known William after he came home and was perhaps directly familiar with the family's famous sword. Such an injury might also explain why William turned his energies to serving on public health committees and newspaper and real estate business ventures when he came home in 1861, rather than returning to a medical practice that would require manual dexterity; see "Defied the Peruvian Troops: She Spread the Stars and Stripes on The Steps and Dared Them to Cross It" [obituary], *Springfield* [Mass.] *Republican* (March 1, 1896): 8. The story is noted as taken from *The Ohio State Journal.*

50. A newspaper report from Panama on June 18, 1859, names "Mr. Trevitt, formerly Consul at Valparaiso . . . on his way to the United States" among the passengers landing in Panama on the steamship *Washington*—which had left Valparaiso on May 29. The steamer was then sailing for San Francisco, after dropping its East-Coast-bound passengers in Panama in order to make the trip east across the isthmus to ships that would sail north up the Atlantic to New York. *Daily Alta California,* July 3, 1859, p. 4. President James Buchanan's official nomination of William Trevitt to fill the consular vacancy in Callao, Peru, is dated in the Congressional record to January 23, 1860. *Journal of the Executive Proceedings of the Senate of the United States* 11 (January 24, 1860): 127.

51. On the accounts about the hospital immediately after the Trevitts were forced out of the consulate, a letter from the Valparaiso correspondent dated February 22, 1860, and published in *The New York Times* on April 11, 1860, notes,

> Day before yesterday (Monday 19th) Dr. Trevitt, for-
> merly consul for the United States at this port, sailed for
> Callao . . . The hospital remains in charge of Dr. Sawyer,

who is employed as surgeon on board the Fredonia. The hospital has been removed from the former premises of Dr. Page, to a cottage in one of the back streets, in the ravine of San Francisco, a building owned by Mr. Riobo. Neither for commodiousness nor for salubrity [sic] of situation can it be compared with the spot on which, for so many years, it has been located, and from which it has been so unnecessarily removed.

"From Chile: Washington's Birthday at Valparaiso, the Indians['] Relations with the United States Varieties," *The New York Times*, April 11, 1860. Six months later, the Valparaiso correspondent provided an update, writing, "The American Hospital has passed into the hands of Dr. A. Reid. Dr. Sawyer, who has had charge of it since Consul Trevitt's removal to Callao, is to leave shortly." "Items of American Interest from Chili [sic]," *The New York Times*, November 5, 1860. See further below on Dr. Reid (Ried).

52. For the original secretary of state correspondence on how the US government ultimately chose to address Chile's cancellation of Trevitt's *exequatur*, see John Bassett Moore, *A Digest of International Law* (Washington, DC: Government Printing Office, 1906), vol. 2, §297, pp. 787–91. For details about William Trevitt's government expenses in Chile, see United States Senate, Committee on Commerce, 43rd Congress, Session 1, Report No. 161, March 6, 1874; and United States Government Documents, *The Executive Documents, printed by order of the House of Representatives During the Second Session of the 42nd Congress, 1871–72*, 18 vols. (Washington, DC: Government Printing Office, 1872), vol. 6, "Executive Document no. 11, Names of Consular Agents and Amounts Paid," pp. 160–72 [=pp. 545–53 in the digital document]. This latter document, an auditor's report from De Benneville Randolph Keim, "Agent of the United States" to George S. Boutwell, secretary of the Treasury in Washington 1871, contains a scathing account of bookkeeping under William's administration. Through the details of Keim's report, we learn that government-funded

"relief" expenses included medical care, food, clothing, shelter, and burial costs. Keim describes the relief account books from Trevitt's tenure as: "kept very badly in lead pencil . . . the most disgraceful I have yet seen, and if it does not indicate downright dishonesty, the amounts are so incredible and inconsistent, that I cannot believe they were expended under a strict observance of the law . . . [an] extraordinary exhibition of liberality at the expense of the Government" (pp. 169–70). An abridged version of Keim's report is also available in *Reports of De B. Randolph Keim, Agent of the United States, Etc., to the Secretary of the Treasury, Relating to the Condition of the Consulates of the United States in Japan, China, Cochin China, Malay Peninsula, Java, British India, Egypt, and on the East and West Coasts of South America* (Washington, DC: Government Printing Office, 1871), 119–22.

53. David Trumbull, *Journals*, Princeton Theological Seminary Library, The David and Jane Wales Trumbull Manuscript Collection, Series 1 (bound journals); Trumbull's entries for December 29, 1858, and March 8, 1859, are in Box 3:2.

54. Jane Trumbull, *Journals*, Princeton Theological Seminary Library, The David and Jane Wales Trumbull Manuscript Collection, Series 8, Box 11. Jane's journal entries, available only up to 1852 and after 1868, do not include the Trevitts' time in Chile.

55. His name is sometimes spelled Reid in newspaper reports, but Trumbull consistently identified him as Ried in his journal entries. Dr. James Aquinas Ried, who took over the American Hospital in the fall of 1860, was a German-speaking immigrant who studied medicine in Great Britain before moving to Valparaiso in 1844; he died in Chile in 1869 and may have been one of the doctors at the German Hospital; see e.g., Adolfo Reccius, *Das deutsche Krankenhaus in Valparaiso, und seine Zeit: Deutsche Artze in Chile* (Santiago: Deutsche-Chilenischen Bund, 1971). For a biography (I have not been able to access it), see Franz Fonck, "Dr. Aquinas Ried: Lebensbild eines Deutschen in Chile," in Carlos Keller, ed., *Dr. Aquinas Ried: Leben und*

Werke (Santiago: Verlag des wissenschaftlichen Archivs von Chile, 1927), 1–64.

56. In a *New York Times* story from November 2, 1861, the Valparaiso correspondent wrote, "Our first American physician, Dr. Page, (who has had the hospital for invalid seamen for many years, but from whose care these were withdrawn by Consul Trevitt) has recently offered the new Consul to receive the patients at seventy-five cents a day, instead [of] $1.25 a day, as now paid.... Dr. Page has hospital premises which he purchased for the purpose of accommodating the United States patients, and for two years these premises have been lying unoccupied, while the invalid seamen have been kept in inferior accommodations because of cheaper rent. . . ." "From Valparaiso," *New York Times*, December 8, 1861, http://www.nytimes.com/1861/12/08/news/valparaiso-political-amnesty-continuation-comm ercial-embarrassments-santiago.html, accessed 2/21/14.

57. David Trumbull, Valparaiso, March 18, 1863 letter published in *Thirty-fifth Annual Report of the American Seamen's Friend Society* (New York: S. Halley, Book & Job Printer, 1863), 32. James Muller's letter of June 1864 was published in *Thirty-sixth Annual Report of the American Seamen's Friend Society* (New York: S. Halley, Book & Job Printer, 1864), 33.

58. Prue Draper, "Thomas Stokes Page," *RootsWeb*, http://wc.rootsweb.ancestry.com/cgi-bin/igm.cgi?op=GET&db=:2516 223&id=I325, accessed 2/15/14.

59. De B. Randolph Keim, to George S. Boutwell, United States Government Documents, Executive Document no. 11, "Names of Consular Agents and Amounts Paid," 1871, 171.

60. Nicholas Senn, "Travel Notes from South America," *Journal of the American Medical Association* 50, no. 1 (January 4, 1908), 37.

61. *Franklin County at the Beginning of the Twentieth Century* (Columbus: Historical Publishing Company, 1901), 188 on "Cholera in the Penitentiary."

62. As evidenced by William's 1846 letter to Henry from Cincinnati, described above.

63. Ohio General Assembly House of Representatives, *Journal of the House of Representatives of the General Assembly of the State of Ohio: Being the Second Session of the Fifty-Second General Assembly, commencing on Monday, January 5, 1857, (Being the Fourth Session under the New Constitution)*, vol. 53 (Columbus: Richard Nevins, State Printer, 1857), Special Report of the Standing Committee on the Penitentiary, In "Appendix to House Journal for the Year 1857," p. 96.

64. *Ohio State University College of Medicine Graduates, 1836–1968* (Columbus: Ohio State University Libraries), 669, https://hsl.osu.edu/sites/hsl.osu.edu/files/Graduates.pdf, accessed 2/25/14.

65. Fort Wayne Genealogy Center Reference Librarian John D. Beatty documents Henry's three weeks as an itinerant daguerreotype photographer at the hotel-tavern, the Hedekin House, in Fort Wayne, Indiana, in April 1848, in John D. Beatty, *Directory of Fort Wayne Photographers 1843–1930*, n.p., under "Trevitt," http://www.genealogycenter.org/pdf/DirectoryofFortWaynePhotographers.pdf, accessed 5/10/14. Fort Wayne was not far from land that William owned in nearby Williams County, Ohio.

66. Reference in the 1850 Columbus City business directory to Henry Trevitt as a "Daguerreian" photographer (boarding with Dr. William Trevitt) is found in *The New Daguerreian Journal* 2, no. 3 (May 1974), 19, http://www.cdags.org/cdags_resources/ndj_02_03.pdf, accessed 2/25/14. The U.S. Census of September 19, 1850, which lists him as "Henry Treavitt," notes his reported occupation as "Artist," living in the household of Dr. William Trevitt and family.

67. The earliest possible date for their engagement is based on the watch's inscribed patent date of June 15, 1858, though it could possibly have been purchased as early as December 1857. The date of her death and all else about her remain unknown to me.

68. The son who was psychologically traumatized by the fire seems most likely to have been William's oldest son, John Noble, who was seventeen at the time, since the newspaper report had blamed it on "too much study," suggesting an adolescent with known dedicated study habits. Of William's other sons, Carlos

was only sixteen months, Butler six, and Willie fifteen. It cannot be Willie since Charles Rand's account of the consular siege mentions him actively helping his parents to resist the soldiers. Willie was also the only son who would stay with his father in Peru the following year, and who was known throughout his adult life for his skills in foreign languages, later going into the newspaper business; he died of a heart attack at home in Columbus in the late 1880s. The little that is known of John Noble suggests that he was indeed a dedicated student, whose college studies come strangely late in his life, in his twenties and thirties. He is listed as briefly attending Kenyon College in Ohio, among the "non-graduates" of the class of 1869, and in 1871 he was a second-year student at Phillips Academy, studying English. He died unmarried, of tuberculosis in May 1875; he was thirty-four. Occasional newspaper references to Butler, who married but had no children and lived only into his late forties, suggest nothing out of the ordinary, though a portrait photo he sent a New Hampshire cousin around 1900 captures a curiously glittering and dazed expression. Carlos, like Henry, held a government job in the Columbus State House as a clerk. He married and had at least one surviving son, Carlos R. Trevitt, who committed suicide on March 27, 1935, purportedly due to the "recent death of near relatives." Ellen Trevitt's address book from the 1930s also notes in a brief entry a "Mrs. Ellison" as "Carlos' daughter," suggesting that the families remained in at least occasional contact.

69. Charles Rand, "Interesting from Valparaiso—Particulars of the attack on the Residence of Dr. Trevitt, the American Consul." On the news of their "nearly restored" health, see "Dr. Wm. Trevitt," *Daily Ohio Statesman*, 5, no. 267 (April 10, 1859): 2, citing "private advice from Valparaiso" via the *Ashland Democrat* and dated March 23. On the fate of the six men arrested on March 4, we know only that Bartolome Riobo was indeed sentenced to death "among others of the Revolutionary Party" ("Latest South American News," *New York Evening Express*, June 9, 1859, n.p.) One short history of Chile in 1859 suggests that the charges for many revolutionary leaders were ultimately commuted to

temporary banishment (André Cochut, *Chile in 1859*. Translated from the *Revue des Deux Mondes* [n.p., 1859], at p. 47). The French photographer Eugenio Maunoury has left a visual records of Valparaiso in 1859 and 1860, including at least one of prisoners captured and chained to logs while awaiting execution in 1860, http://www.allposters.com/-sp/Condemned-to-Death-Valparaiso-Chile-circa-1860-Posters_i1589477_.htm, accessed 5/10/14.

70. John Martyn Harlow, the physician who treated Gage during his unexpected recovery, published the case as "Passage of an Iron Rod through the Head," *Boston Medical and Surgical Journal*, December 13, 1848, reprinted in *Journal Neuropsychiatry* 11, no. 2 (1999): 281–83.

71. See, e.g., Malcolm MacMillan, *An Odd Kind of Fame: Stories of Phineas Gage* (Cambridge: MIT Press, 2002). Dr. MacMillan's research has generated a flurry of media attention on Gage, including discovery of two daguerreotypes, one included in this chapter. Following Gage's death in California, with his family's permission, Harlow obtained Gage's skull and the iron rod, both now on display at Harvard Medical School. I thank Dr. MacMillan and his research assistant, Matthew L. Lena, for communication about Henry's witness to meeting Gage in Chile.

72. Henry's report of Gage at the medical meeting was soon published in the *Ohio Medical and Surgical Journal* 13, no. 2 (November 1, 1860), 173, reprinted in the *Boston Medical and Surgical Journal* no. 1709; 63, no. 16 (November 15, 1860): 327. We know nothing about how this recognition of Henry in the Boston medical literature might have helped his reputation as a doctor when he returned to New England. The story was reprinted much later (mistakenly calling Henry a resident of Cincinnati) in G. Archie Stockwell, "Brain Wounds with Excessive Loss of Structure," *Therapeutic Gazette* 13, series 3, 5, no. 4 (April 15, 1889): 232–37, at 237.

73. We learn of William's bankruptcy from an 1877 legal case in which William sued for his wife Lucinda's right to retain a tract of land in northwest Ohio that William had

purchased in 1841 (he says as a trust for her based on a verbal agreement between them) with funds she brought to their marriage in 1839. For documentation of this 1841 purchase (including Lucinda's name), see Weston Arthur Goodspeed and Charles Blanchard, *County of Williams, Ohio: Historical and Biographical, with an Outline Sketch of the Northwest Territory, of the State, and Miscellaneous Matters* (Chicago: F. A. Battey & Co., 1882), 315–16. The 1877 case ruled in Lucinda's favor even though married women had not gained a legal right to own property until 1861. The suit was clearly a desperate attempt on the couple's part to hold onto what they could, given that "On the tenth day of January, 1877, Trevitt made a general assignment of all his property, real and personal, for the benefit of his creditors." (Sessions vs. Trevitt, *The Ohio Law Journal*, 4 [September 25, 1883]; see also E. L. Dewitt, *Reports of Cases Argued and Determined in the Supreme Court of Ohio*, N.S. 39 [New York: Banks and Brothers, Law Publishers, 1884], 259–68). A newspaper account of the public auction in 1878, which notes that "The bidding was dull and the sales very low," also reveals that "Dr. William Trevitt's residence. . .was purchased by John Trevitt, nephew of the Doctor, of New Hampshire, for $6,310." (*Daily Ohio State Journal* 39, no. 214, September 9, 1878: 1). Like Henry, John—who in fact spent over $11,000 that day to help rescue his uncle's real estate—would spend the rest of his life in New Hampshire, but his intervention in this crisis clearly saved William and Lucinda from homeless penury. William's obituary three years later notes that he "died at his residence." ("Death of Dr. Trevitt, News from Columbus," *Cincinnati Commercial Tribune* 41, no. 142, February 9, 1881: 1). On John Trevitt's capture at New Orleans in the Civil War, see *Biographical Review 23: Containing Life Sketches of Leading Citizens of Hillsboro and Cheshire Counties, New Hampshire* (Boston: Biographical Review Publishing Co., 1897), 67.

74. "Report of County Commissioners." *The Farmers' Cabinet* 67, no. 42, May 6, 1869.

75. Dr. Samuel Gridley Howe, *Third Annual Report of the Massachusetts Board of State Charities* (Boston: 1867), lix, cited in F. B. Sanborn, *Supplement to the Twelfth Annual Report: The Public Charities of Massachusetts during the Century Ending Jan. 1, 1876: A Report Made to the Massachusetts Centennial Commission, February 1, 1876*, Board of State Charities Public Document No. 17 (Boston: Wright and Potter State Printers, 1876), cxix.

76. Henry Trevitt, court testimony in the case against Elwin Major, as quoted in *Nashua Daily Telegraph*, Nashua, New Hampshire, September 18, 1875, p. 2. Henry reported that when he had left Ida after her delivery, "I saw nothing to lead me to believe that the third child would not live. When I returned it was in a dying condition." See also Milli S. Knudsen, *Hard Times in Concord, New Hampshire: The Crimes, the Victims, and the Lives of the State Prison Inmates 1812-1883* (Westminster, MD: Heritage Books, 2008). For the medical details of Ida's poisoning, see Robert Amory and Edward S. Wood (eds.), *Wharton and Stille's Medical Jurisprudence*, Fourth Edition (Philadelphia: Kay and Brother, 1884), Vol. 2, §597-98, "Case XLIV: Poisoning by Strichnine (From the Report of the Trial of Edwin [sic] W. Major)." Shortly before he was hanged, Major wrote a letter (later published in the local papers) to his two surviving children, a boy and a girl who then disappear from history. I am grateful to Milli S. Knudsen, historian and genealogist, for her kind assistance in locating the Nashua newspaper reports and other related details about the trial and the family.

77. Mrs. Davison of Wilton, court testimony as published in the *New Hampshire Patriot*, (September 22, 1875), 3.

78. J. A. Swaney, July 19, 1861, a letter published in the *33rd Annual Report of the American Seamen's Friend Society* (New York: S. Halley, Book & Job Printer, 1861), 33: "Dr. Trevitt, our present U.S. Consul, takes an interest in our church, and attends services regularly with his family."

79. After her marriage Ellen was often known as "Ellenor" (with variant spellings) to distinguish her from John's wife Ellen, her sister-in-law in nearby Mont Vernon; I have called her Ellen

throughout this chapter to maintain consistency with her birth record as well as the 1850 census. The elderly clergyman who married Ellen and Henry is commonly referred to in most sources as Unitarian but self-identifies in the 1870 census as "Cong[regationalist]." Written public records (including census records) suggest that Ellen's mother consistently avoided identifying her Catholic background or her parents' immigration to Canada from Ireland in 1820, although the facts are stated clearly enough on their tombstone in the old St. Patrick's Catholic cemetery high on a windy hill overlooking the bay in Digby, Nova Scotia. I am grateful to Karen Ellis Russell for copies of the birth and census records pertaining to Ellen Trevitt, Holly Cobb for access to (and permission to quote from) the childhood journals and letters of Henry's oldest daughter, Carita (1875–1906), and the late Ruth Holman for notes on Wilton town tax records documenting Henry's earnings as a physician to the county poor.

80. Carita Trevitt to Will Cushman, unpublished letter, April 30, 1900.

Chapter 4

1. Avi Shlaim, "Four Days in Seville," ElPais.com, September 9, 2004, http://users.ox.ac.uk/~ssfc0005/Four%20Days%20in%20 Seville.html, accessed 2/25/14.

2. Daniel Barenboim, as quoted in Elena Cheah, *An Orchestra Beyond Borders: Voices of the West-Eastern Divan Orchestra* (London: Verso, 2009), vii.

3. Daniel Barenboim, as quoted in Cheah, *An Orchestra Beyond Borders*, viii.

4. As quoted by Daniel Cohen, in Cheah, *An Orchestra Beyond Borders*, 13.

5. Daniel Cohen, in Cheah, *An Orchestra Beyond Borders*, 13–14.

6. Sumner B. Twiss, "Religion and Human Rights: A Comparative Perspective," The B. Frank Hall Memorial Lecture, University of North Carolina at Wilmington, Feb. 22, 1996, unpublished manuscript, 6. I thank Professor Twiss for sharing this

manuscript with me, and for granting me the privilege to explore my early ideas about human rights language in patristic sources as a participant in the 1996 American Academy of Religion Roundtable Session he co-sponsored with Professor Arvind Sharma on "Religion and Human Rights."

7. Sumner B. Twiss, "Religion and Human Rights: A Comparative Perspective," 5.

8. Nicholas Kristof, "Evangelicals without Blowhards," *New York Times* blog post, July 30, 2011, http://www.nytimes.com/2011/07/31/opinion/sunday/kristof-evangelicals-without-blowhards.html?_r=0, accessed 2/25/14.

9. Paul E. Farmer, as quoted in Mary Frances Schjonberg, "Raise Prophetic Voices against Poverty, Paul Farmer tells Bishops: Medical Anthropologist Underscores Importance of Achieving MDGs," *Episcopal News Service*, Sept. 21, 2007, http://archive.episcopalchurch.org/79901_90263_ENG_HTM.htm, accessed 8/18/14.

10. Paul E. Farmer, "Three Stories, Three Paradigms, and a Critique of Social Entrepreneurship: Remarks Delivered at the Skoll World Forum 2008," in Paul E. Farmer, *To Repair the World: Paul Farmer Speaks to the Next Generation* (Berkeley: University of California Press, 2013), 40. Partners In Health, the non-governmental organization (NGO) that Farmer helped to co-found, is one example of a global community driven by a human rights perspective to economic and health needs. As one of his former students puts it, "Farmer never sees his work as service. He sees it as solidarity"; as quoted in Katie Koch, "Family Values, in an Orphanage: At the Divinity School, Soni built on a Service Ethos that Spans Generations," *Harvard Gazette*, May 24, 2012. http://news.harvard.edu/gazette/story/2012/05/a-legacy-well-served/, accessed 5/25/12.

11. Johannes Morsink, *The Universal Declaration of Human Rights: Origins, Drafting, and Intent* (Philadelphia: University of Pennsylvania, 2000), 192.

12. This is the focus of, for example, John Nurser's study on Fred Nolde, *For All People and All Nations: Christian Churches*

and Human Rights (Geneva: World Council of Churches Publications, 2005).

13. For further discussion, see, e.g., Thomas Pogge, "Severe Poverty as a Violation of Negative Duties," *Ethics and International Affairs* 19, no. 1 (2005): 55–84.

14. The Universal Declaration of Human Rights is widely available in print and online in more than four hundred languages. Official sources and translations are available from the United Nations Office of the High Commission for Human Rights, http://www.ohchr.org, accessed 11/15/10.

15. "Third-generation rights," not discussed here, are those today called "cultural rights," such as the rights of a particular ethnic group to maintain its own native language and cultural practices.

16. Micheline R. Ishay, *The History of Human Rights: From Ancient Times to the Globalization Era* (Berkeley: University of California Press, 2004).

17. Mary Ann Glendon, *A World Made New: Eleanor Roosevelt and the Universal Declaration of Human Rights* (New York: Random House, 2001); Johannes Morsink, *The Universal Declaration of Human Rights: Origins, Drafting and Intent* (Philadelphia: University of Pennsylvania, 2000); and Johannes Morsink, *Inherent Human Rights: Philosophical Roots of the Universal Declaration* (Philadelphia: University of Pennsylvania Press, 2009); See also Ishay, *The History of Human Rights*, esp. 16–18 and 211–29.

18. This summary is derived from the online history of the United Nations, at http://www.un.org/en/aboutun/history/, accessed 11/15/10.

19. Known as the "Four Freedoms Speech." Further information and historical audio archives are at http://www.fdrlibrary. marist.edu/fourfreedoms, accessed 4/1/11.

20. In discussion of political law and governance, nations are often referred to as nation states, or "States"; the word is capitalized to emphasize a united government entity. United Nations members are often referred to as "member States."

21. The World Bank, and its origin in meetings at Bretton Woods, New Hampshire, will not be discussed in this book. The World Bank has been much criticized for its role as a lending agency that many believe condones corruption and traps poor nations in a strangling spiral of debt. See, e.g., Kevin Danaher, ed., *Fifty Years Is Enough: The Case Against the World Bank and the International Monetary Fund* (Boston: South End Press, 1999); and Dambisa Moyo, *Dead Aid: Why Aid Is Not Working and How There Is a Better Way for Africa* (New York: Farrar, Straus and Giroux, 2010).

22. For Humphrey's account of the UDHR's creation and meetings through to the final vote, see John P. Humphrey, *Human Rights and the United Nations: A Great Adventure* (Dobbs Ferry, NY: Transnational Publishers, 1984); John P. Humphrey, *On the Edge of Greatness: The Diaries of John Humphrey, First Director of the United Nations Division of Human Rights. Volume 1, 1948-1949*, ed. A. J. Hobbins, Fontanus Monograph Series 4 (Montreal: McGill University Libraries, 1994). Hereafter noted as "Humphrey, *Diaries*."

23. Humphrey, *Diaries*, 48 (September 27, 1948): "My mind is completely open to the question of God's existence: I neither believe nor disbelieve."

24. On Cassin, see Glenda Sluga, "René Cassin: *Les droits de l'homme* and the Universality of Human Rights, 1945-1966," in *Human Rights in the Twentieth Century*, ed. Stefan-Ludwig Hoffman (New York: Cambridge University Press, 2010), 107-24. Humphrey wrote on Cassin, "His faults are small ones, his qualities great." (Humphrey, *Diaries*, 90 [December 8, 1948]). According to Morsink (*The Universal Declaration*, 194), Cassin was at first reluctant to treat ESC rights as full legal rights on the same level with civil rights. Historian Jay Winter has recently described Cassin's lifelong dedication to supporting Jewish education and social justice through his leadership of the Alliance Israelite Universelle; Jay Winter, "Réne Cassin and the Alliance Israélite Universelle," *Modern Judaism* 32, no. 1 (2012): 1-21.

25. Ishay, *The History of Human Rights*, 17.

26. On Maritain, see Andrew Woodcock, "Jacques Maritain, Natural Law and the Universal Declaration of Human Rights," *Journal of the History of International Law* 8 (2006): 245–66. On his earlier thought related to political action, see Jacques Maritain, "Catholic Action and Political Action," Chapter 8 in Maritain's *Scholasticism and Politics* (New York: The MacMillan Co., 1940), 194–224.

27. Humphrey, *Diaries,* 83 (November 22, 1948), on Articles 25 and 26.

28. Humphrey, *Diaries,* 81 (November 20, 1948).

29. Humphrey, *Diaries,* 39 (September 8, 1948).

30. Article 25.2 was originally Article 34 in the Commission's Second Session; for more detail, see Morsink, *The Universal Declaration,* 195–96 and 257–58.

31. Although 25(1) uses only masculine pronouns and 25(2) concerns only women and children, the UDHR, like most documents from its era, uses masculine pronouns with a generic intent to include both men and women.

32. Morsink, *The Universal Declaration,* 258.

33. Morsink, *The Universal Declaration,* 191–238, esp. 191–210. What follows here substantially draws on this section from Morsink.

34. On the history of the contested nature of second- and third-"generation" rights, see also Peter Uvin, *Human Rights and Development* (Bloomfield, CT: Kumarian Press, 2004), esp. 38ff; for René Cassin's role in shaping this distinction from the tripartite French motto, "Liberté, égalité, fraternité," see Ishay, *The History of Human Rights,* 18ff. For more about the controversies over ESC rights, see, e.g., Alicia Ely Yamin, "The Future in the Mirror: Constructing and De-Constructing Strategies for the Defense and Promotion of Economic, Social and Cultural Rights," *Human Rights Quarterly* 27, no. 3 (2005): 1200–44; and Alicia Ely Yamin, "Reflections on Defining, Understanding and Measuring Poverty in Terms of Violations of Economic and Social Rights Under International Law," *Georgetown Journal on Fighting Poverty* 4 (1997): 273–307.

35. On this view, see, e.g., Michael Ignatieff, *Human Rights as Politics and Idolatry*, ed. Amy Gutmann (Princeton: Princeton University Press, 2001); and Samuel Moyn, *The Last Utopia: Human Rights in History* (Cambridge, MA: Harvard University Press, 2010).

36. In this context, we should also remember that even those countries that signed their agreement to the UDHR and thus have taken a principled position of agreement with its wording on ideal rights for all, need not abide by it in strict legal terms since the UDHR is not a legally binding document.

37. Morsink, *The Universal Declaration*, 192.

38. Morsink, *The Universal Declaration*, 192.

39. For the relevance of the right to health to the United States, see Alicia Ely Yamin, "The Right to Health under International Law and Its Relevance to the United States," *American Journal of Public Health* 95, no. 7 (2005): 1156–61.

40. Morsink, *The Universal Declaration*, 193.

41. Morsink, *The Universal Declaration*, 197.

42. For discussion of these various attempts to revise Article 22 and Article 25 into a more obvious harmony that would avoid repetition, see Morsink, *The Universal Declaration*, 204–08.

43. Morsink, *The Universal Declaration*, xi.

44. Humphrey, *Human Rights and the United Nations: A Great Adventure*, 75.

45. Morsink, *The Universal Declaration*, xi–xii, citing Hurst Hannum, "The Status of the Universal Declaration of Human Rights in National and International Law," *Georgia Journal of International and Comparative Law*, 25, nos. 1–2 (1995/1996): 287–397.

46. Morsink, *The Universal Declaration*, 284.

47. Morsink, *The Universal Declaration*, 285.

48. Morsink, *The Universal Declaration*, 286.

49. Quoted in Morsink, *The Universal Declaration*, p. 288, note 17.

50. The literature on the Covenants is immense. Two representative summaries are David Beetham, "What Future for Economic and Social Rights?" *Political Studies* 43 (1995): 41–60; and Stephen P. Marks, "The Past and Future of the Separation of Human

Rights into Categories," *Maryland Journal of International Law* 24 (2009): 208–43.

51. ICESCR Article 11.2 (b), http://www.ohchr.org/EN/Professional Interest/Pages/CESCR.aspx, accessed 4/15/11.

52. There are of course many unofficial documents, manuals, and guidelines that also attempt to spell out and interpret the ICESCR in a way that will make a real difference for real people in advancing social justice and positive health. As one of many examples, a practical guide to economic, social, and cultural rights that is designed for use by health-care workers in resource-limited settings is that of Partners In Health, "Addressing the Social Determinants of Health," Unit 11 in Partners In Health, *Program Management Guide* (Boston: PIH, 2011), http://www.pih.org/library/pih-program-management-guide/unit-11-addressing-t he-social-determinants-of-health, accessed 11/14/11.

53. See, e.g., http://www.ohchr.org/EN/Issues/Health/Pages/SRRightHealthIndex.aspx (Special Rapporteur on the Right to Health); and http://www.srfood.org/en (Special Rapporteur on the Right to Food). See now Jean Ziegler, Christophe Golay, Claire Mahon, and Sally-Anne Way, *The Fight for the Right to Food: Lessons Learned*, International Relations and Development Series (London: Palgrave Macmillan, 2011).

54. http://www.echr.coe.int/Documents/Convention_ENG.pdf, accessed 11/14/11.

55. http://www.hrcr.org/docs/Banjul/afrhr.html, accessed 11/14/11.

56. http://acerwc.org/the-african-charter-on-the-rights-and-welfare-of-the-child-acrwc/, accessed 11/14/11.

57. http://legal.un.org/avl/ha/catcidtp/catcidtp.html, accessed 11/14/11.

58. http://www.ohchr.org/EN/ProfessionalInterest/Pages/CERD.aspx, accessed 11/14/11.

59. http://www.ohchr.org/en/professionalinterest/pages/crc.aspx, accessed 11/14/11.

60. http://www.un.org/disabilities/convention/conventionfull.shtml, accessed 11/14/11.

61. http://www.un.org/womenwatch/daw/cedaw/, accessed 11/14/11.

62. Peter Walker, Dyan Mazurana, Amy Warren, George Scarlett, and Henry Louis, "The role of spirituality in humanitarian crisis

survival and recovery," in *Sacred Aid: Faith and Humanitarianism*, ed. Michael Barnett and Janice Gross Stein (New York: Oxford University Press, 2012), 131. This story is, of course, not actually about human rights but rather about respect for religion as part of principled action that supports ESC rights-related issues.

63. He tells the story in Bas de Gaay Fortman and Jacques Paul Klein, *Peace in the 21st Century: Between the Supranational and the Grassroots* (Wageningen, the Netherlands: Educatief Centrum 'Hotel De Wereld,' 2000), 5–17.

64. Bas de Gaay Fortman, *Political Economy of Human Rights: Rights, Realities, and Realization*; Routledge Frontiers of Political Economy (London & New York: Routledge, 2011), 129.

65. Fortman, *Political Economy of Human Rights*, 129–30.

66. Fortman, *Political Economy of Human Rights*, 128.

67. "The Russian Orthodox Church's Basic Teaching on Human Dignity Freedom and Rights, Bishops' Council of the Russian Orthodox Church, 2008 (Osnovy 2008), IV.8, http://www. mospat.ru/ru/documents/dignity-freedom-rights/, as cited in Alfons Brüning and Evert van der Zweerde, eds, *Orthodox Christianity and Human Rights*, Eastern Christian Studies 13 (Leuven: Peeters Publishers, 2012), 280.

68. Alasdair MacIntyre, *After Virtue* (Notre Dame, IN: University of Notre Dame Press, 1981), 67.

69. See especially Esther D. Reed, *The Ethics of Human Rights: Contested Doctrinal and Moral Issues* (Waco, TX: Baylor University Press, 2007), esp. 167–74; Ethna Regan, *Theology and the Boundary Discourse of Human Rights* (Washington, DC: Georgetown University Press, 2010); and Nicholas Wolterstorff, *Justice: Rights and Wrongs* (Princeton, NJ: Princeton University Press, 2008). On Wolterstorff's personal views on justice and rights, see also now Nicholas P. Wolterstorff, *Journey Toward Justice: Personal Encounters in the Global South* (Grand Rapids, MI: BakerAcademic, 2013).

70. Wolterstorff, *Justice: Rights and Wrongs*, 331.

71. Roger Ruston, *Human Rights and the Image of God* (London: SCM Press, 2004), 13.

72. Nicholas Wolterstorff, "The Way to Justice: How My Mind Has Changed," *Christian Century*, December 1, 2009, 26–30, at 29.

73. Nicholas Wolterstorff, *Justice: Rights and Wrongs*, 62. While Wolterstorff clearly supports a rights model, his careful thinking and appeal for more conservative Christians may mean that his recent work on social justice and "agapism" could offer an alternative way of thinking for those who still quail at the thought of talking in church about human rights; for Wolterstorff on agapism see now Nicholas Wolterstoff, *Justice in Love*, Emory University Studies in Law and Religion (Grand Rapids: Eerdmans, 2011). I thank the Rev. Joslyn Ogden Schaefer for this observation.

74. I thank Laura Alexander for the observation outlined in this paragraph. On Clement of Alexandria, see, for example, Annewies van den Hoek, "Widening the Eye of the Needle: Wealth and Poverty in the Works of Clement of Alexandria," in *Wealth and Poverty in Early Church and Society*, ed. Susan R. Holman, Holy Cross Studies in Patristic Theology and History (Grand Rapids, MI: BakerAcademic/Holy Cross Greek Orthodox Press, 2008), 67-75.

75. Gregory of Nazianzus, *Or.* 14.24; for translation, see Martha Vinson, trans., *St. Gregory of Nazianzus: Select Orations* (Washington, DC: Catholic University of America Press, 2003), 39-71; and Brian Daley, S. J., *Gregory of Nazianzus*, The Early Church Fathers (New York: Routledge, 2006), 76-97.

76. Asterius of Amasea, *hom.* 3.12.3; for the Greek, see the critical edition of C. Datema, *Asterius of Amasea: Homilies I-XIV: Text, Introduction and Notes* (Leiden: E. J. Brill, 1970), 35, lines 11-14.

77. On this view in Basil of Caesarea, see discussion in Susan R. Holman, "Healing the World with Righteousness? The Language of Social Justice in Early Christian Homilies," in *Charity and Giving in Monotheistic Religions*, ed. Miriam Frenkel and Yaacov Lev, Studien zur Geschichte und Kultur des islámischen Orients (Berlin: De Gruyter, 2009), 89-110; this essay is a more developed examination of research that first took shape in an earlier article, "The Entitled Poor: Human Rights Language in the Cappadocians," *Pro Ecclesia* 9 (2000): 476-89. For the Cappadocians' general focus on social justice and civic identity, see Susan R. Holman, *The Hungry are Dying: Beggars*

and Bishops in Roman Cappadocia (New York: Oxford University Press, 2001).

78. All translations here come from Anthony Bowen and Peter Garnsey, ed./trans., *Lactantius: Divine Institutes*, Translated Texts for Historians (Liverpool, UK: Liverpool University Press, 2004). I thank Luke Bretherton for inspiring me to reexamine Lactantius.

79. Lactantius, *Divine Institutes* 5.14.9, ed./trans. Bowen and Garnsey, 309-10. Peter Phan's translation gives this as "equity"; Peter C. Phan, *Social Thought*, Message of the Fathers of the Church 20 (Wilmington, DE: M. Glazier, 1984), 96.

80. Lactantius, *Div. Inst.* 5.14.16-17, selections, ed./trans. Bowen and Garnsey, 310, my emphasis.

81. Lactantius, *Div. Inst.* 5.14.20, ed./trans. Bowen and Garnsey, 311.

82. Lactantius, *Div. Inst.* 5.15.4, ed./trans. Bowen and Garnsey, 311.

83. Here quoting Wolterstorff, *Justice: Rights and Wrongs*, 22.

84. Lactantius, *Div. Inst.* 6.10.2, ed./trans. Bowen and Garnsey, 349.

85. Lactantius, *Div. Inst.* 6.11.17-19, selections, ed./trans. Bowen and Garnsey, 354. The teaching that those who can help but do not are guilty of murder is one that recurs in later patristic texts as well. Basil of Caesarea, for example, writes in his homily *In Time of Famine and Drought* (8.7) that "whoever has the ability to remedy the suffering of others, but chooses rather to withhold aid out of selfish motives, may properly be judged the equivalent of a murderer"; C. Paul Schroeder, trans., *St Basil the Great: On Social Justice*, Popular Patristic Series (Crestwood, NY: St. Vladimir's Seminary Press, 2009), 85.

86. Lactantius, *Div. Inst.* 6.11.28, ed./trans. Bowen and Garnsey, 355.

87. Lactantius, *Div. Inst.* 6.12.39, ed./trans. Bowen and Garnsey, 359.

88. Lactantius, *Div. Inst.* 3.13.12, ed./trans. Bowen and Garnsey, 190.

89. Bowen and Garnsey, introduction to Lactantius *Div. Inst.*, 2.

90. Codex Theodosianus (hereafter CT) 11.27.1, trans. Clyde Pharr, *The Theodosian Code and Novels and the Sirmondian*

Constitutions (Princeton: Princeton University Press, 1952, reprinted New York, 1969), 318. While somewhat peripheral to a discussion of economic and social rights in antiquity, readers interested in learning more about the authorship controversies over Pharr's translation may wish to consult Linda Jones Hall, "Clyde Pharr, the Women of Vanderbilt, and the Wyoming Judge: The Story behind the Translation of the Theodosian Code in Mid-Century America," *Roman Legal Tradition* 8 (2012): 1–42, http://romanlegaltradition.org/contents/2012/RLT8-JONESHALL.PDF, accessed 8/25/14.

91. CT 11.27.2, trans. Pharr, 318.
92. Pharr, *The Theodosian Code*, 388–89; The comment about socialized medicine is in note 1.
93. CT 16.2.42, trans. Pharr, 448.
94. CT 16.2.43, trans. Pharr, 448.
95. *Theod. Novel Val. Title 12*, in Pharr, 526.
96. Discussed at length in, e.g., Moshe Weinfeld, *Social Justice in Ancient Israel and in the Ancient Near East* (Jerusalem: Hebrew University Magnes Press, 1995).
97. CT 14.18.1, in Pharr, 420.
98. I have explored examples and implications of these differences in Susan R. Holman, "Out of the Fitting Room: Rethinking Patristic Social Texts on 'The Common Good'," in *Reading Patristic Texts on Social Ethics: Issues and Challenges for Twenty-First-Century Christian Social Thought*, ed. Johan Leemans, Brian Matz, and Johan Verstraeten (Washington: Catholic University of America Press, 2011), 103–23.
99. This story and all quotes that follow are taken from Alicia Ely Yamin, "Rights-Based Approach to Health," the Ivan and Janice Stone Lecture, Beloit College, Beloit, Wisconsin, November 17, 2010, https://www.youtube.com/watch?v=Pd-WREXfr9A, accessed 8/25/14. See also Alicia Ely Yamin, *Power and Suffering: Human Rights-Based Approaches to Health and Why They Matter* (Philadelphia: University of Pennsylvania Press, forthcoming). For a broader context to the human rights discussion in this conflict, see Alicia Ely Yamin, "Protecting and Promoting the Right to Health in Latin America: Selected

Experiences from the Field," *Health and Human Rights: An International Journal* 5, no. 1 (2000): 117–48. For more on Yamin's personal journey, see also Alicia Ely Yamin, "Health and Human Rights in Latin America and Beyond: A Lawyer's Experience with Public Health Internationalism," in *Comrades in Health: U.S. Health Internationalists, Abroad and at Home*, ed. Anne-Emanuelle Birn and Theodore M. Brown (New Brunswick, NJ: Rutgers University Press, 2013), 238–53.

100. See, e.g., Alicia Ely Yamin and Siri Gloppen, eds., *Litigating Health Rights: Can Courts Bring More Justice to Health?* (Cambridge, MA: Harvard University Press, 2011).

101. Rowan Williams, "Shaping Holy Lives," in *The Oblate Life*, ed. Gervase Holdaway (Collegeville, MN: Liturgical Press, 2008), 152.

Chapter 5

1. I thank James R. Cochrane, Jill Olivier, and Teresa Cutts for their comments on earlier drafts of this chapter. It should be noted that I have no affiliation with ARHAP and the views I express in this chapter do not necessarily represent those of the researchers engaged in this collaborative consortium; any remaining factual errors here are wholly mine.

2. Leymah Gbowee, "It's Time to End Africa's Mass Rape Tragedy," *The Daily Beast*, April 5, 2010, http://www.thedailybeast.com/articles/2010/04/05/its-time-to-end-africas-mass-rape-tragedy.html, accessed 1/18/14.

3. "Address by the Minister of Social Development, Ms. Bathabile Dlamini MP on the occasion of the National Inter-Faith Summit," November 29, 2013, http://www.dsd.gov.za/index.php?option=com_content&task=view&id=554&Itemid=82, accessed 1/18/14.

4. Readers interested in more information might begin with John W. de Gruchy, with Steve de Gruchy, *The Church Struggle in South Africa, 25th Anniversary Edition* (Minneapolis: Fortress Press, 2005); and Tracy Kuperus, "The Political Role and

Democratic Contribution of Churches in Post-Apartheid South Africa," *Journal of Church and State* 53, no. 2 (2011): 278–306.

5. Janet Heard, "Kotze's 'Priceless Gem' Honored," *Cape Times*, February 8, 2013, http://www.iol.co.za/capetimes/theo-kotze-s-priceless-gem-honoured-1.1466500#.UtsS2Sj0DJw, accessed 1/18/14.

6. On Kotze's appointment as Sobukwe's chaplain, see Benjamin Pogrund, *How Can Man Die Better . . . Sobukwe and Apartheid* (London: Peter Halben, 1990), 270–71. Considering how radical Kotze was, Pogrund notes (270) it was surprising "that the Department of Prisons accepted him as a chaplain; it must have been a mistake." For the story of Theo Kotze's life and ministry, see Jean Knighton-Fitt, *Beyond Fear* (Cape Town: PreText Publishers, 2003).

7. On Beyers Naudé, see, e.g., Colleen Ryan, *Beyers Naudé: Pilgrimage of Faith* (Grand Rapids: Eerdmans, 1990).

8. Nelson Mandela, "Speech by President Nelson Mandela at the celebration of Beyers Naudé's 80th Birthday," May 23, 1995, http://www.anc.org.za/show.php?id=3550, accessed 2/11/14.

9. James R. Cochrane, "Agapé: The Cape Office of the Christian Institute," *Journal of Theology for Southern Africa* 118 (March 2004): 58, 61.

10. Jim Cochrane, "In Memory of Theo Kotze, a South African of Courage," Memorial address at the Rosebank Methodist Church, Cape Town, July 15, 2003, p. 3, https://www.academia.edu/1680555/In_Memory_of_Theo_Kotze_a_South_African_of_Courage, accessed 12/19/13.

11. James R. Cochrane, personal communication, 2/3/14.

12. John de Gruchy, "Foreword," in James R. Cochrane, *Circles of Dignity: Community Wisdom and Theological Reflection* (Minneapolis: Fortress Press, 1999), viii. Information on Kotze and Cochrane in this paragraph is drawn from Jim Cochrane, "In memory of Theo Kotze"; Theologian Frances Young, whom Kotze and his wife befriended in Birmingham, remembered his life as an "exile through the wilderness" that impressed her with "a sense that the global and individual dimensions of human life are not separate, but mirrored in one another."

Frances M. Young, *Brokenness and Blessing: Towards a Biblical Spirituality* (Grand Rapids: Baker Academic, 2007), 33; "Rondebosch United Church: Our Ministers Past and Present," http://www.rondeboschunited.org.za/history/our-ministers-p ast-and-present, accessed 1/1/14; and James R. Cochrane, "Agapé: The Cape Office of the Christian Institute," 53–68.

13. Steve de Gruchy, "Reinhold Niebuhr and South Africa," *Journal of Theology for Southern Africa* 80 (September 1992): 24–38, at p. 24.

14. Steve de Gruchy, "Curriculum Vitae: April 2008," http://sorat.ukzn.ac.za/Libraries/Sorat_Staff_CVs/cv_s_degruchy_ April08.sflb.ashx, accessed 10/19/13. Those who sought religious conscientious objector (CO) status in South Africa during apartheid had a much more difficult experience than those in the United States who sought CO status during the Vietnam War. Laws in South Africa made conscientious objection, even on religious grounds, often frankly illegal unless one belonged to a historically consistent pacifist group (e.g., the Quakers), or (as was the case for Steve de Gruchy) one had the resources (and government permission) to argue one's case in court and could clearly demonstrate that one's convictions were consistent and separate from politics. Faced with such barriers, many men simply failed to sign up and either left the country or spent time in prison. For more information, see, e.g., Richard L. Abel, *Politics by Other Means: Law in the Struggle against Apartheid, 1980–1994* (New York: Routledge, 1995), 67–124; Daniel Conway, *Masculinities, Militarisation and the End Conscription Campaign: War Resistance in Apartheid South Africa* (Manchester, UK and New York: Manchester University Press/Palgrave Macmillan, 2012); and Gary Thatcher, "South Africa's Conscientious Objectors: A Long Fight by a Nation's Pacifists," *Christian Science Monitor*, September 4, 1980; http://www.csmonitor.com/1980/0904/090469.html, accessed 1/18/14.

15. James R. Cochrane, "Steve de Gruchy—In Memoriam." *Practical Matters* 4 (Spring 2011): 2, http://practicalmattersjournal.

org/sites/practicalmattersjournal.org/files/pdf/issue2/de%20 Gruchy_FINAL.pdf, accessed 9/13/13.

16. Desmond Tutu, "God Is God's Worst Enemy: The First Steve de Gruchy Memorial Lecture" (Congregational Church, Rondebosch, South Africa, April 24, 2012), 1.

17. Beverley Haddad, "Steve de Gruchy (1961–2010)" [Obituary], *Natalia* 40 (2010): 146–47, http://www.pmbhistory.co.za/ portal/witnesshistory/custom_modules/Supplement_PDFs/ Steve_De_Gruchy.pdf, accessed 9/13/13.

18. My primary sources for the life of Steve de Gruchy include: S. M. de Gruchy, "Curriculum vitae: April 2008"; Steve de Gruchy, "Reversing the Biblical Tide: What Kuruman Teaches London about Mission in a Post-Colonial Era," *Acta Theologica Supplementum* 12 (2009): 48–62; Steve de Gruchy, "A Symphony in Stone: Leadership, Vocation and the State's Attack on Tiger Kloof School," *Journal of Theology for Southern Africa* 118 (March 2004): 100–13; Beverley Haddad, "Steve de Gruchy (1961–2010);" Tinyiko Sam Maluleke, "A tribute to Steve de Gruchy," *Ecumenical Water Network*, March 4, 2010, http://water.oikoumene.org/en/whatwedo/news-events/a-tribute-to-steve-de-gruchy, accessed 1/1/14; "Steve de Gruchy's Life Celebrated," *The Witness*, March 1, 2010, http://www.witness.co.za/index.php?showcontent&global%5B_id%5D=36612, accessed 1/1/14; Desmond Tutu, "God Is God's Worst Enemy"; and Denise M. Ackerman, "Steve de Gruchy: A Legacy of Risk, Resistance and Hope," Second Steve de Gruchy Memorial Lecture, March 20, 2013, http://christianspirit.co.za/2013/04/02/2nd-steve-de-gruchy-memorial-lecture-by-prof-denise-m-ackermann/, accessed 1/1/14. See also now John W. de Gruchy, *Led Into Mystery: Seeking Answers in Life and Death* (London: SCM Press, 2013).

19. For more about the Lesotho mission, see Tim Couzens, *Murder at Morija: Faith, Mystery, and Tragedy on an African Mission*, Reconsiderations in Southern African History (Charlottesville, VA: University of Virginia Press, 2005).

20. John P. Kretzman and John L. McKnight, *Building Communities from the Inside Out: A Path Toward Finding and Mobilizing a*

Community's Assets (Chicago: ACTA Publications. 1993). All quotes in this paragraph are from p. 7.

21. The ABCD concepts were among the nuanced dynamics that helped to inform, for example, the extraordinary work of church-based neighborhood revitalization in Sandtown, an inner-city neighborhood of Baltimore, described in Mark R. Gornik, *To Live in Peace: Biblical Faith and the Changing Inner City* (Grand Rapids: Eerdmans, 2002). See also Steve Corbett and Brian Fikkert, *When Helping Hurts: How to Alleviate Poverty Without Hurting the Poor and Yourself* (Chicago: Moody Press, 2009), esp. Chapter 5, "Give me your Tired, your Poor, and their Assets" (125–39). A related concept is "Appreciate Inquiry"; its influence on development efforts in mission settings is described in Bryant Myers, *Walking with the Poor: Principles and Practices of Transformational Development*, revised edition (Maryknoll, New York: Orbis, 2011).

22. For the asset-based approach, see Kretzmann and McKnight, *Building Communities from the Inside Out*; for Steve's early reflections on the use of this approach in South Africa, see Steve de Gruchy, "Of Agency, Assets and Appreciation: Seeking Some Commonalities Between Theology and Development," *Journal of Theology for Southern Africa* 117 (2003): 20–39.

23. "Steve de Gruchy's life celebrated," *The Witness*. The paper was Steve de Gruchy, "Dealing with Our Own Sewage: Spirituality and Ethics in the Sustainability Agenda," Address to the World Conference on Theologies of Liberation, Belem, Brazil, January 2009. http://archived.oikoumene.org/fileadmin/ files/wcc-main/documents/p4/ewn/resource_database/ deGruchy%20WFTL_paper.pdf, accessed 1/1/14.

24. http://academic.sun.ac.za/theology/jointconference/Confe rence%20Programme1.pdf, accessed 1/1/14.

25. For more about Snow and Whitehead, see Steven Johnson, *The Ghost Map: The Story of London's Most Terrifying Epidemic— and How It Changed Science, Cities, and the Modern World* (New York: Riverhead Books, 2006). The relationship between this story and ARHAP's work is developed in Gary R. Gunderson and James R. Cochrane, *Religion and the Health*

of the Public: Shifting the Paradigm (New York: Palgrave MacMillan, 2012), esp. 22–26.

26. Steve de Gruchy, "Water and the Spirit: Theology in the Time of Cholera," *World Council of Churches Ecumenical Review* 62, no. 2 (July 2010): 188–201, at 198.

27. *ARHAP International Colloquium: Case Study Focus: Papers and Proceedings, July 2005, Willow Park, Gauteng, South Africa* (Cape Town: ARHAP, 2005), 11–12, http://www.arhap.uct.ac.za/downloads/ARHAP_colloquium2005.pdf, accessed 1/18/14.

28. James R. Cochrane, "Religion, Public Health and a Church for the 21st Century," *International Review of Mission* 95, nos. 376–77 (January 2006): 59–72, at page 62.

29. Gary Gunderson, Deborah McFarland, James R. Cochrane, "Framing Document," as published in *ARHAP International Colloquium: Case Study Focus: July 2005*, 11–12.

30. James R. Cochrane, personal communication, February 3, 2014.

31. "Timeline of the Carter Center," http://www.cartercenter.org/about/history/chronology_1990.html, accessed 9/28/13.

32. http://www.gatesfoundation.org/who-we-are/general-information/leadership/global-health/william-foege, accessed 9/28/13.

33. ARHAP's activities in the United States are discussed further later on in this chapter; see also Miriam Kiser, Deborah L. Jones, Gary R. Gunderson, "Faith and Health: Leadership Aligning Assets to Transform Communities," *International Review of Mission* 95, nos. 376–77 (January/April 2006), 50–58.

34. Gunderson, McFarland, Cochrane, "Framing Document."

35. James R. Cochrane, personal communication, February 3, 2014.

36. Katherine Marshall, "A Discussion with Reverend Canon Ted Karpf," Berkley Center for Religion, Peace & World Affairs, November 13, 2010, http://berkleycenter.georgetown.edu/intervie ws/a-discussion-with-reverend-canon-ted-karpf. All information about Karpf in this chapter is taken from this interview unless noted otherwise.

37. On "3 by 5," see Jim Yong Kim and Charlie Gilks, "Scaling up Treatment—Why We Can't Wait," *New England Journal of Medicine* 353, no. 22 (2005): 2392–94. For a critique of the

initiative, see Paul Benkimoun, "How Lee Yong-wook changed WHO," *The Lancet* 367, no. 9525 (June 3, 2006): 1806–08.

38. Liz Thomas, Barbara Schmid, Malibongwe Gwele, Rosemond Ngubo, and James R. Cochrane, '*Let us Embrace*': *The role and significance of an integrated faith-based initiative for HIV and AIDS* (Rondebosch, South Africa, and Atlanta, Georgia: African Religious Health Assets Programme, 2006), 16, http://www.arhap.uct.ac.za/downloads/masang_full.pdf, accessed 9/13/13. All information in this chapter about Masangane is taken from this report.

39. Thomas et al., *Let us Embrace*, 9.

40. Thomas et al., *Let us Embrace*, 19 and 44.

41. For more on CHWs, including the importance of paying them, see Partners In Health, "Strengthening human resources," Unit 5 in *Program Management Guide* (Boston: Partners In Health, 2011), 136–63, http://www.pih.org/library/pih-program-management-guide/unit-5-strengthening-human-resources, accessed 1/18/14; and Prabhjot Singh and Dave A. Chokshi, "Community Health Workers: A Local Solution to a Global Problem" [perspective] *New England Journal of Medicine* 369 (September 5, 2013): 894–96, DOI: 10.1056/NEJMp1305636, accessed 1/18/14.

42. Thomas et al., *Let us Embrace*, 28.

43. Thomas et al., *Let us Embrace*, 32.

44. http://www.ems-online.org/uploads/media/2013-05-05_Report_South_Africa_2013_01.pdf, accessed 10/22/13.

45. The 2006 report includes extensive details about the PIRHANA tool set, including correspondence, permissions forms, and questionnaires: http://www.arhap.uct.ac.za/pub_WHO2006.php, accessed 2/14/14.

46. James R. Cochrane, personal communication, February 3, 2014.

47. The German Institute for Medical Mission (Difaem) and the World Council of Churches, for example, used it for research in Ghana, Kenya, and Malawi; Beate Jakob, "Assessing and Mobilizing Religious Health Assets in Christian Settings: Interim Report on a Study Conducted by Difaem and WCC," presentation at ARHAP Conference, "When religion

and health align," July 2009, Cape Town, http://www.arhap. uct.ac.za/downloads/Wed_Jakob_prez.pdf (presentation); http://www.arhap.uct.ac.za/downloads/Wed_Jakob_paper.pdf (working paper), accessed 1/1/14.

48. For another description of intangible assets, see Wilkinson-Maposa et al., *The Poor Philanthropist*, 3 vols (Cape Town: UCT Graduate School of Business, 2006 [vol. 1] and Cape Town: Southern Africa-United States Center for Leadership and Public Values, 2009 [vols. 2–3]).

49. Vesper Society, "Gifted by God in the Mission of Health and Well-Being: An Interview with Steve de Gruchy," *VeNews*, September 2006, http://www.vesper.org/newsletter/2006_09_ venews.shtml, accessed 1/1/14.

50. Denise M. Ackermann, "Steve de Gruchy: A legacy of risk, resistance and hope."

51. African Religious Health Assets Programme (ARHAP). *ARHAP International Colloquium: Case Study Focus*, 2005, 46–47.

52. Paul Germond told this story in a lecture at Emory University, "Healthworlds: Conceptualizing Landscapes of Health and Healing," Religion and Public Health Collaborative, December 2, 2009. See also Paul Germond and James R. Cochrane, "Healthworlds: Conceptualizing Landscapes of Health and Healing," *Sociology* 44 (2010): 307–24; and James R. Cochrane, "The Language that Difference Makes," *Practical Matters* 4 (Spring 2011): 1–16, esp. 10–13.

53. Lucy Gilson, "The Relevance of Healthworlds to Health System Thinking about Access," in *When Religion and Health Align: Mobilizing Religious Health Assets for Transformation*, ed. James R. Cochrane, Barbara Schmid, and Teresa Cutts (Dorpspruit, South Africa: Cluster Publications, 2011), 164–77, at 169.

54. Thomas et al., *Let us Embrace*, 71, n. 206, summarizing an early draft of the Germond-Cochrane paper.

55. Gary Gunderson, "The Missing Space," in *FaithHealth: A Magazine of the Division of Faith and Health Ministries, Wake Forest Baptist Health*, Wake Forest, North Carolina: Wake Forest Baptist Health, Spring 2013, p. 2.

56. Jill Olivier, James R. Cochrane, and Barbara Schmid, with Lauren Graham, *ARHAP Bibliography: Working in a Bounded Field of Unknowing* (Cape Town, South Africa: ARHAP, October 2006). http://www.arhap.uct.ac.za/downloads/arhapbibliog_oct2006. pdf; and Jill Olivier, James R. Cochrane, and Barbara Schmid, with Lauren Graham, *ARHAP Literature Review: Working in a Bounded Field of Unknowing.* Cape Town, South Africa: ARHAP, October 2006, http://www.arhap.uct.ac.za/downloads/ arhaplitreview_oct2006.pdf, both accessed 9/13/13.

57. Beverley Haddad, Jill Olivier, and Steve de Gruchy. *The Potentials and Perils of Partnership: Christian Religious Entities and Collaborative Stakeholders Responding to HIV in Kenya, Malawi and the DRC: Summary Report,* Study commissioned by Tearfund and UNAIDS (Cape Town: ARHAP, 2009), http:// tilz.tearfund.org/~/media/files/tilz/hiv/the%20potentials%20 and%20perils%20of%20partnership.pdf, accessed 9/13/13.

58. Barbara Schmid, Elizabeth Thomas, Jill Olivier, and James R. Cochrane, *The Contribution of Religious Entities to Health in Sub-Saharan Africa,* Study commissioned by Bill & Melinda Gates Foundation (Cape Town: ARHAP, 2008), http://www. arhap.uct.ac.za/pub_Gates2008.php, accessed 9/13/13.

59. African Religious Health Assets Programme (ARHAP). *ARHAP International Colloquium: Case Study Focus,* 2005, 44.

60. What follows in this paragraph is a paraphrase of the eight key conclusions identified in the report.

61. See, e.g., Cochrane, Schmid, and Cutts, *When Religion and Health Align*; Gunderson and Cochrane. *Religion and the Health of the Public*; and James R. Cochrane and Gary R. Gunderson, *The Barefoot Guide to Mobilizing Religious Health Assets for Transformation,* The Third Barefoot Collective. November 2012, http://www.barefootguide.org/barefoot-guide-3.html, accessed 2/25/13.

62. See, e.g., John P. Bartkowski and Helen A. Regis, *Charitable Choices: Religion, Race, and Poverty in the Post-Welfare Era* (New York: New York University Press, 2003). For more on the impact of these government changes on the lives of poor women who self-identified as persons of faith, see Susan Crawford Sullivan,

Living Faith: Everyday Religion and Mothers in Poverty (Chicago: University of Chicago Press, 2011). For a global perspective, although not directly related to religion, see e.g., Arachu Castro and Merrill Singer, eds., *Unhealthy Health Policy: A Critical Anthropological Examination* (Lanham, MD: Altamira Press, 2004). For a recent critique of American government policy as it relates to funding social services for all Americans related to health care, see Elizabeth H. Bradley and Lauren A. Taylor, *The American Health Care Paradox: Why Spending More Is Getting Us Less* (New York: Public Affairs, 2013).

63. "Assessing Religious Health Assets in Two Metro-Atlanta Neighborhoods," *Religion and Health Collaborative* [newsletter], vol. 1, number 1, Spring 2008, p. 1.

64. On "boundary leaders," see Gary Gunderson, *Boundary Leaders: Leadership Skills for People of Faith* (Minneapolis: Fortress Press, 2004); and Gary Gunderson with Larry Pray, *The Leading Causes of Life* (Memphis: Methodist LeBonheur Healthcare, Center of Excellence in Faith and Health, 2006), later published as Gunderson with Pray, *Leading Causes of Life: Five Fundamentals to Change the Way You Live Your Life* (Nashville: Abingdon Press, 2009).

65. Gunderson, "The Other Side of Complexity," 2.

66. Gunderson, "The Other Side of Complexity," 2.

67. Phillip V. Tobias, "Apartheid and Medical Education: The Training of Black Doctors in South Africa," *International Journal of Health Services* 13 (November 1, 1983), 131–53, at 139. Tobias's data on white doctors is from "the late 1970s" and that for black doctors is from 1975 specifically.

68. Gary R. Gunderson, "What do hospitals have to do with health? Exploring the relationships among religious disease care systems and other types of religious health assets," in: *ARHAP International Colloquium, 2007, Collection of Concept Papers*, p. 4.

69. See, e.g., Centers for Disease Control and Prevention, *CDC Health Disparities and Inequalities Report—United States 2013, MMWR* 2013; 62 (*Supplement* 3, pp. 1–187, http://www.cdc.gov/mmwr/pdf/other/su6203.pdf, accessed 1/18/14.

70. See, e.g., Susan M. Reverby, *Examining Tuskegee: The Infamous Syphilis Study and Its Legacy* (John Hope Franklin Series in African American History and Culture; Chapel Hill: University of North Carolina Press, 2009).

71. Source for these numbers and categories: Teresa Cutts, "Mapping Memphis Style: Building & Strengthening a System of Health," Methodist Health Faith & Health, PowerPoint slide presentation, July 18, 2012, http://www.wesleyseminary.edu/ Portals/0/Documents/MVS/TeresaCuttsJuly182012DCDisparity. pdf, accessed 8/18/14. Gunderson has recently noted that the overwhelming majority of volunteer liaisons in the Memphis program are women, usually women who have a paying job in a helping or health-care profession. Rev. Dr. Gary Gunderson, "Navigating the Affordable Care Act," lecture at Garrett Evangelical Theological Seminary, October 1, 2013, https://www. youtube.com/watch?v=viowu6Lv9eM, accessed 8/25/14.

72. David Dault, "Congregations and Health: An Interview with Dr. Teresa Cutts and Rev. Bobby Baker," *Things Not Seen* radio podcast #1219, November 11, 2012, http://www. thingsnotseenradio.com/1219-congregations-and-health/#. Uts4Qyj0DJw, accessed 1/18/14.

73. Cutts and Gunderson as quoted in Alex Halperin, "It Really Does Take a Village: How Memphis is Fixing Healthcare," *Salon. com*, September 3, 2013, http://www.salon.com/2013/09/03/ it_really_does_take_a_village_how_memphis_is_fixing_ healthcare/, accessed 1/18/14.

74. Agency for Healthcare Research and Quality (AHRQ), "Church-Health System Partnership Facilitates Transitions from Hospital to Home for Urban, Low-Income African Americans, Reducing Mortality, Utilization, and Costs," AHRQ Health Care Innovations Exchange, March 14, 2012, http://www.pnamidsouth.org/images/content/Cutts.pdf, accessed 10/7/14; See also Gary R. Gunderson and Teresa Cutts, "Protestant congregations: Aligning and leveraging assets for vulnerable populations and governmental partners who care for them," Paper commissioned by Urban Strategies, LLC, Arlington, VA. Memphis: Methodist LeBonheur Healthcare

Center of Excellence in Faith and Health, Summer 2011, http://www.methodisthealth.org/dotAsset/40dac89a-987d-4799-b39a-aedb83ccc286.pdf, accessed 10/28/13.

75. "Leading Causes of Life," news item in *FaithHealth: A Magazine of the Division of Faith and Health Ministries, Wake Forest Baptist Health* (Wake Forest, North Carolina: Wake Forest Baptist Health, Spring 2013), 13.

76. See, e.g., Bradley and Taylor, *The American Health Care Paradox.*

77. Bradley and Taylor, *The American Health Care Paradox*, 17.

78. For more on what's needed to close this global health care delivery gap, see also Rose Calnin Kagawa, Andrew Anglemyer, and Dominic Montagu, "The Scale of Faith Based Organization Participation in Health Service Delivery in Developing Countries: Systematic Review and Meta-Analysis," *PLoS One* 7, no. 11 (November 2012), doi: e48457, http://www.plosone.org/article/info%3Adoi%2F10.1371%2Fjournal.pone.0048457, accessed 10/28/13. Rachel Mash and Robert Mash, "Faith-Based Organizations and HIV Prevention in Africa: A Review," *African Journal of Primary Health Care Family Medicine* 5, no. 1 (2013), http://dx.doi.org/10.4102/phcfm.v5i1.464; Jill Olivier and Quentin Wodon, eds., *Strengthening the Evidence for Faith-Inspired Health Engagement in Africa*, 3 vols., HNP Discussion Paper Series (Washington, DC: The World Bank, 2012), http://documents.worldbank.org/curated/en/docsearch/report/76223, accessed 10/28/13; See also Rolando L. Santiago, "Faith-Based Organizations and Public Health," in *Igniting the Power of Community: The Role of CBOs and NGOs in Global Public Health*, ed. P. A. Gaist (New York: Springer, 2010), 93–108.

79. James Cochrane, "Steve de Gruchy—In Memoriam," 2.

80. See especially de Gruchy, "Of Agency, Assets and Appreciation."

81. African Religious Health Assets Programme (ARHAP). *ARHAP International Colloquium 2007: Monkey Valley Resort, Cape Town, South Africa, March 13–16, 2007, Collection of Concept Papers*, Cosponsored by Methodist Healthcare, University of Cape Town, Vesper Society, and Emory University, both at p. 155.

82. Fiona Scorgie, *ARHAP's International colloquium 2007, Collection of Concept Papers*, 149.

83. Jo Wreford, "Worlds Apart? Religious Interpretations and Witchcraft in the Negotiations of Health Strategies for HIV/AIDS in South Africa," African Religious Health Assets Programme, *Assessing and Mobilizing Religious Health Assets in Christian Settings: Interim Report on a Study Conducted by Difaem and WCC. When Religion and Health Align: Mobilizing Religious Health Assets for Transformation, ARHAP Conference, Cape Town, 13-16 July 2009*, http://www.arhap.uct.ac.za/downloads/Wed_Wreford_paper.pdf, accessed 1/1/14.

84. On justice, see, e.g., James R. Cochrane, "Fire from Above, Fire from Below: Health, Justice and the Persistence of the Sacred," *Theoria* 55, no. 116 (August 2008): 67–96; and James R. Cochrane, "The Incommensurability of Development and Justice," in *Living on the Edge: Essays in Honour of Steve de Gruchy, Activist and Theologian*, ed. James R. Cochrane, Elias Bongmba, Isabel Phiri, and Des van der Water (Pietermaritzburg, South Africa: Cluster Publications, 2012), 188–200.

85. James R. Cochrane, personal communication, February 3, 2014. For further discussion on this social nature of the claim to rights, particularly in the South African context, see Laurie Ackermann, *Human Dignity: Lodestar for Equality in South Africa* (Claremont, South Africa: Juta and Co. Ltd., 2012).

86. Steve de Gruchy, "Taking Religion Seriously: Some Thoughts on 'Respectful Dialogue' Between Religion and Public Health in Africa," in *ARHAP International Colloquium 2007: Collection of Concept Papers*, Cape Town, March 13-16, 2007 (Cape Town: ARHAP, 2007), pp. 7–11, http://www.arhap.uct.ac.za/downloads/ARHAP_colloquium2007.pdf, accessed 9/24/13. What follows in here is my paraphrase of de Gruchy's main points.

Chapter 6

1. Amy Goodman, "*Tè Tremblé*: Journey to the Epicenter," Democracy Now! news video interview, Jan. 22, 2010, http://www.democracynow.org/2010/1/22/t_trembl_journey_to_the_epicenter, accessed 3/10/10.

2. See Kim Ives, "Massive Earthquake Wreaks Devastation in Haiti," *Haiti Liberté* 3, no. 26 (January 13-19, 2010), online at

http://www.haiti-liberte.com/archives/volume3-27/Massive%20
Earthquake%20Wreaks%20Devastation%20in%20Haiti.asp,
accessed 3/10/10. Goodman also mentions the incident and
community response in Amy Goodman and Denis Moynihan,
*The Silenced Majority: Stories of Uprisings, Occupations,
Resistance, and Hope* (Chicago: Haymarket Books, 2012), 259.

3. Tukufu Zuberi, "Has Foreign Aid Hurt Haiti? An Interview
with Mario Joseph," *Huffington Post*, April 6, 2012, http://
www.huffingtonpost.com/dr-tukufu-zuberi/mario-
joseph-haiti_b_1392750.html, accessed 12/19/13.

4. C. S. Lewis, *The Four Loves* (audio CD) (Nashville: Thomas
Nelson, 2004). The passage given here is not in Lewis's book of
the same title but is found only in the radio talk, recorded in
London by the Episcopal Radio-TV Foundation in 1958.

5. Marcel Mauss, *The Gift: The Form and Reason for Exchange
in Archaic Societies*, ed. W. D. Hall (New York: W. W. Norton,
1990), with a foreword by Mary Douglas; and Margaret Visser,
The Gift of Thanks: The Roots and Rituals of Gratitude (Boston:
Houghton Mifflin Harcourt, 2009). See also Michael Satlow,
ed., *The Gift in Antiquity*, The Ancient World: Comparative
Histories (Malden, MA: Wiley-Blackwell, 2013). A number
of excellent studies on the gift from the perspectives of
anthropology and philosophy are available that press far
beyond the narrow focus of themes explored in this book;
see, e.g., John D. Caputo and Michael J. Scanlon, eds., *God,
The Gift, and Postmodernism* (Bloomington, IN: Indiana
University Press, 1999, influenced by Jacques Derrida's *Given
Time 1: Counterfeit Money*, trans. Peggy Kamuf [Chicago:
University of Chicago Press, 1992]); Marcel Hénaff, *The
Price of Truth: Gift, Money, and Philosophy*, trans. Jean-Louis
Morhange with the collaboration of Anne-Marie Feenberg-
Dibon (Stanford: Stanford University Press, 2010); Jean-Luc
Marion, *Being Given: Toward a Phenomenology of Givenness*,
trans. Jeffrey L. Kosky (Stanford: Stanford University Press,
2002); and Kathryn Tanner, *Economy of Grace* (Minneapolis:
Augsburg Fortress Press, 2005). I thank Crina Gschwandtner

for the references related to the gift and postmodern philosophy.

6. Steve de Gruchy, "Of Agency, Assets and Appreciation: Seeking Some Commonalities between Theology and Development," *Journal of Theology for Southern Africa* 117 (November 2003): 20-39, at 37.

7. http://www.fns.usda.gov/wic/women-infants-and-children-wic, accessed 2/20/14. For an evaluation of WIC's effectiveness in improving the health of its participants, see David Rush, "The National WIC Evaluation: Evaluation of the Special Supplemental Food Program for Women, Infants, and Children," *American Journal of Clinical Nutrition* 48, no. 2 (1988): 389-519.

8. One much-cited contemporary model is that of conditional cash transfers (CCT), government-supported electronic fund transfers that may be tied to health-related behaviors such as clinic visits and school attendance. There are many debates over how CCTs can work most effectively. The best known example is that of Mexico's Oportunidades program; see, e.g., Tina Rosenberg, "Helping the World's Poorest, for a Change," *The New York Times*, January 7, 2011, http://opinionator. blogs.nytimes.com/2011/01/07/helping-the-worlds-poorest-for-a-change/?_php=true&_type=blogs&_r=0, accessed 2/22/14. See also Beryl Lieff Benderly, "A Bargain or a Burden? How Conditional Cash Transfer (CCT) Program Design Affects the Women Who Participate in Them," *Results-Based Financing for Health* (New York: The World Bank, March 2011), https://www.rbfhealth.org/news/item/477/ bargainburdencctprogramdesignaffectswomen, accessed 2/22/14; and Paul Gertler, "Do Conditional Cash Transfers Improve Child Health? Evidence from PROGRESA's Control Randomized Experiment," *The American Economic Review* 94, no. 2 (2004): 336-41. On the power of women's literacy to improve their children's health even if they are very poor and their schooling was of terrible quality, see now Robert A. LeVine, Sarah LeVine, Beatrice Schnell-Anzola, Meredith L. Rowe, and Emily Dexter, *Literacy and Mothering: How*

Women's Schooling Changes the Lives of the World's Children (New York: Oxford University Press, 2012).

9. Ann Swidler and Susan Cotts Watkins, "'Teach a Man to Fish': The Sustainability Doctrine and Its Social Consequences," *World Development* 37, no. 7 (2009): 1182–96; all quotes in the discussion that follows here about this study are from page 1192.

10. David R. Loy, "The Poverty of Development: Buddhist Reflections," *Development* 46, no. 4 (2003): 7–14, at p. 13.

11. Daryl Collins, Jonathan Murduch, Stuart Rutherford, and Orlanda Ruthven, *Portfolios of the Poor: How the World's Poor Live on $2 a Day* (Princeton, NJ: Princeton University Press, 2009).

12. Deepa Narayan with Raj Patel, Kai Schafft, Anne Rademacher, and Sarah Koch-Schulte, eds., *Voices of the Poor: Can Anyone Hear Us?* (Washington, DC, and New York: Oxford University Press for the World Bank, 2000) [Vol. 1]; Deepa Narayan, Robert Chambers, Meera Kaul Shah, Patti Petesch, eds., *Voices of the Poor: Crying out for Change* (Washington, DC, and New York: Oxford University Press for the World Bank, 2000) [Vol. 2]; and Deepa Narayan and Patti Patesch, eds., *Voices of the Poor: From Many Lands* (Washington, DC, and New York: Oxford University Press for the World Bank, 2002)[vol. 3]. Summarizing their findings in the *Voices of the Poor* series, for example, the authors wrote, "What they need, the poor said over and over, was the dignity of work, fair treatment, a living wage, and not handouts." Narayan et al., *Voices of the Poor* 1: 36.

13. Ruth Levine and the What Works Working Group, with Molly Kinder, *Millions Saved: Proven Successes in Global Health* (Washington, DC: Center for Global Development, 2004), updated in Ruth Levine, *Case Studies in Global Health: Millions Saved* (Burlington, MA: Jones and Bartlett, 2007).

14. http://www.transparency.org/country, accessed 8/25/14.

15. The African Religious Health Assets Programme under contract to the World Health Organization, *Appreciating Assets: The Contribution of Religion to Universal Access in Africa: Mapping, Understanding, Translating, and Engaging Religious Health Assets in Zambia and Lesotho in Support of Universal Access to*

HIV/AIDS Treatment, Care and Prevention (Cape Town, South Africa: ARHAP, October 2006), 68.

16. Jean-Pierre Habicht, "Malnutrition Kills Directly, Not Indirectly," [letter] *The Lancet* 371, no. 9626 (2008): 1749–50; and R. E. Black, L. H. Allen, Z. A. Bhutta, L. E. Caulfield, M. de Onis, M. Ezzati, C. Mathers, J. Rivera, for the Maternal and Child Undernutrition Study Group, "Maternal and Child Undernutrition: Global and Regional Exposures and Health Consequences," *The Lancet* 371, no. 9608 (2008): 243–60.

17. Food and Agriculture Organization of the United Nations, *The State of Food Insecurity in the World: Economic Growth Is Necessary But Not Sufficient to Accelerate Reduction of Hunger and Malnutrition* (Rome: Food and Agriculture Organization of the United Nations, 2012), 9, Table 1. Annual reports are available online at http://www.fao.org/publications/sofi/en/, accessed 2/22/14.

18. Jamie Bartram and Sandy Cairncross, "Hygiene, Sanitation, and Water: Forgotten Foundations of Health," *PLoS Medicine* 7, no. 11 (2010): e1000367, http://www.plosmedicine.org/article/info:doi/10.1371/journal.pmed.1000367.

19. African Religious Health Assets Programme, *Appreciating Assets*, 62.

20. Erica Bornstein, "Religious Giving Outside the Law in New Delhi," in *Sacred Aid: Faith and Humanitarianism*, ed. Michael Barnett and Janice Gross Stein (New York: Oxford University Press, 2012), 140–65, esp. 143–44. Derrida also examines the idea of the "divine economy" in the Christian tradition, in Jacques Derrida, *The Gift of Death*, trans. David Wills (Chicago: University of Chicago Press, 1995).

21. Mary Douglas, "No Free Gifts," Foreword to Mauss, *The Gift*, vii.

22. Aafke Elisabeth Komter, "Gratitude and Gift Exchange" in *The Psychology of Gratitude*, ed. Robert A. Emmons and Michael E. McCullough (New York: Oxford University Press, 2004), 207. Komter identifies the poet as Marina Tsvatajeva; I have used here the more common English spelling.

23. Kim Ives, "Massive Earthquake Wreaks Devastation in Haiti."

258 | NOTES TO PAGES 180-181

24. See, e.g., Margaret Visser, *The Gift of Thanks: The Roots and Rituals of Gratitude* (New York: Houghton Mifflin Harcourt, 2009); Aafke E. Komter, *Social Solidarity and the Gift* (New York: Cambridge University Press, 2005); David Steindl-Rast, "Gratitude as Thankfulness and as Gratefulness," in *The Psychology of Gratitude*, 282–89; and Komter, "Gratitude and Gift Exchange" in *The Psychology of Gratitude*, 195–212.
25. Gregg E. Gardner, "Charity Wounds: Gifts to the Poor in Early Rabbinic Judaism," in Satlow, ed., *The Gift in Antiquity*, 173–88.
26. Tzvi Novick, "Charity and Reciprocity: Structures of Benevolence in Rabbinic Literature," *Harvard Theological Review* 105, no. 1 (2012): 33–52.
27. See, e.g., Moshe Weinfeld, *Social Justice in Ancient Israel and in the Ancient Near East* 36 (Jerusalem and Minneapolis: The Hebrew University Magnes Press and Fortress Press, 1995). For modern views on the relationship between justice and mercy as it may relate to religious discussion, see, e.g., Martha C. Nussbaum, "Equity and Mercy," *Philosophy and Public Affairs* 22 (1993): 83–125; Krister Stendahl, "Judgment and Mercy," in *The Context of Contemporary Theology: Essays in Honor of Paul Lehmann*, ed. Alexander J. McKelway and E. David Willis (Atlanta: John Knox Press, 1974), 147–54; and Jacob Neusner, "The Theological Category-Formations of Rabbinic Midrash: [3]: God's Justice and God's Mercy," in idem, *The Theological Foundations of Rabbinic Midrash* (Lanham, MD: University Press of America, 2006), 63–89. I thank Sarah Coakley for these references.
28. See, e.g., "The Heroic Deeds of Mar Rabbula," in *Stewards of the Poor: The Man of God, Rabbula, and Hiba in Fifth-Century Edessa*, trans. Robert Doran, Cistercian Studies Series 208 (Kalamazoo, MI: Cistercian Publications, 2006), 90. For more on the language of social justice in health-care initiatives for the poor in late antiquity, see Susan R. Holman, "Healing the world with righteousness? The Language of Social Justice in Early Christian Homilies," in *Charity and Giving in Monotheistic Religions*, ed. Miriam Frenkel and Yaacov Lev, Studien zur Geschichte und Kultur des islamischen Orients (Berlin and New York: De Gruyter, 2009), 89–110.

29. Stendahl, "Judgment and Mercy," 148–49.
30. On widows' prayers (and their identification as "altar"), see, e.g., the *Didascalia Apostolorum* (sometimes dated to the third century), in R. Hugh Connolly, trans., *Didascalia Apostolorum* (Oxford: Clarendon Press, 1929, repr. 1969), 88, 133–34, 143, 156; Connolly's translation is the most complete; an earlier translation based only on the Syriac manuscript, translated in 1903 by Margaret Dunlop Gibson (London: C. J. Clay and Sons) is available online at https://archive.org/details/didascaliaaposto00gibsuoft, accessed 8/25/14. On the role of widows in the early church, see also Bonnie Bowman Thurston, *The Widows: A Women's Ministry in the Early Church* (Minneapolis: Fortress Press, 1989). For further discussion about patristic views on gifts and loans for the poor, including those who are sick, see, e.g., Susan R. Holman, *The Hungry are Dying: Beggars and Bishops in Roman Cappadocia* (New York: Oxford University Press, 2001); Helen Rhee, *Loving the Poor, Saving the Rich: Wealth, Poverty, and Early Christian Formation* (Grand Rapids: BakerAcademic, 2012); and Brenda Ihssen, *'They Who Give From Evil:' The Response of the Eastern Church to Money-Lending in the Early Christian Era* (Eugene, OR: Wipf and Stock, 2012).
31. Daniel F. Caner, "Alms, Blessings, Offerings: The Repertoire of Christian Gifts in Early Byzantium," in Satlow, ed., *The Gift in Antiquity*, 25–44.
32. Caner, "Alms, Blessings, Offerings," 29.
33. On exchanges within economically poor communities, see, e.g., Susan Wilkinson-Maposa, Alan Fowler, Ceri Oliver-Evans, and Chao F. N. Mulenga, *The Poor Philanthropist: How and Why the Poor Help Each Other* (Cape Town: UCT Graduate School of Business, 2006). Subsequent volumes included Wilkinson-Maposa and Fowler, *The Poor Philanthropist II: New Approaches to Sustainable Development* (Cape Town: Southern Africa-United States Center for Leadership and Public Values, 2009) and Susan Wilkinson-Maposa for the Community Grantmaking and Social Investment Programme, Southern Africa-United States Centre for Leadership and Public Values, *The Poor Philanthropist III: A Practice-Relevant Guide for*

Community Philanthropy (Cape Town: Southern Africa-United States Center for Leadership and Public Values, 2009).

34. LiErin Probasco, *More Good than Harm: Moral Action and Evaluation in International Religious Volunteer Tourism*, PhD Diss., Princeton University, 2013. See especially her Chapter 7, "Recipient Perspectives on Interpreting Aid." I thank Dr. Probasco for sharing her work with me.

35. Probasco, *More Good than Harm*, 242.

36. Probasco, *More Good than Harm*, 243.

37. Probasco, *More Good than Harm*, 322–26.

38. See, e.g., Michael Maren, *The Road to Hell: The Ravaging Effects of Foreign Aid and International Charity* (New York: The Free Press, 1997); Linda Polman, *Crisis Caravan: What's Wrong with Humanitarian Aid?*, trans. Liz Waters (New York: Metropolitan Books, 2010); and Timothy T. Schwarz, *Travesty in Haiti: A True Account of Christian Missions, Orphanages, Food Aid, Fraud, and Drug Trafficking* (Lexington, KY: BookSurge Publishing, 2008).

39. Cardinal Francis George, OMI, Catholic Archbishop of Chicago, "Catholic Social Teaching and Economic Globalization," Public lecture for the Religions & Public Life Series, The Kenan Institute for Ethics at Duke University, February 12, 2013.

40. Paul Pierre, "Lessons from Haiti: Tackling Acute and Chronic Disasters," Remarks made at the 17th Annual Thomas J. White Symposium, Partners In Health, Cambridge, Massachusetts, September 25, 2010; See also Paul Pierre, "Moral Responsibility in a Context of Scarcity: The Journey of a Haitian Physician," *Narrative Inquiry in Bioethics* 2, no. 2 (Fall 2012): 89–92; Michael Griffin and Jennie Weiss Block, eds., *In the Company of the Poor: Conversations with Dr. Paul Farmer and Fr. Gustavo Gutiérrez* (Maryknoll, NY: Orbis Books, 2013); and Roberto S. Goizueta, *Caminemos con Jesús: Toward a Hispanic/Latino Theology of Accompaniment* (Maryknoll, NY: Orbis Books, 2003).

41. Luke Bretherton, *Resurrecting Democracy: Faith, Citizenship and the Politics of a Common Life* (Cambridge: Cambridge University Press, 2014). I thank Dr. Bretherton for sharing this material with me prior to publication. All quotes and references to Bretherton's views here are taken from Chapter 8, "Economy, debt and citizenship."

42. Carlene Bauer, *Frances and Bernard* (Boston: Houghton Mifflin, 2012), 100.

43. Dorothy Day, *The Long Loneliness: An Autobiography* (New York: Harper & Row, 1952), 181.

44. Eric Gregory, "Agape and Special Relations in a Global Economy: Theological Sources," in *Global Neighbors: Christian Faith and Moral Obligations in Today's Economy*, ed. Douglas A. Hicks and Mark Valeri (Grand Rapids: Wm. B. Eerdmans, 2008), 16-42 at 40.

45. Michael Jackson, *Life Within Limits: Well-Being in a World of Want* (Durham, NC: Duke University Press, 2011), 169.

46. Gregory, "Agape and Special Relations in a Global Economy," 42.

47. Lauren Winner, "You might be cooking this very night for people who won't invite you back," *The Hardest Question* [blog], August 26, 2013, http://thq.wearesparkhouse.org/new-testament/lect22cgospel/, accessed 12/24/13.

48. Gustavo Gutiérrez, "Saying and Showing the Poor: 'God Loves You,'" in Griffin and Block (eds.), *In the Company of the Poor*, 32.

Acknowledgments

1. A. G. Sertillanges, *The Intellectual Life*, trans. Mary Ryan (Washington, DC: Catholic University of America Press, 1987), xix.

SELECT BIBLIOGRAPHY

AND SUGGESTIONS FOR

FURTHER READING

Ackermann, Laurie. *Human Dignity: Lodestar for Equality in South Africa*. Claremont, South Africa: Juta and Co. Ltd., 2012.

African Religious Health Assets Program (ARHAP) under contract to the World Health Organization. *Appreciating Assets: The Contribution of Religion to Universal Access in Africa; Mapping, Understanding, Translating, and Engaging Religious Health Assets in Zambia and Lesotho in Support of Universal Access to HIV/AIDS Treatment, Care and Prevention*. Cape Town: ARHAP, October 2006.

African Religious Health Assets Programme (ARHAP). *ARHAP International Colloquium: Case Study Focus: Papers & Proceedings*. Willow Park, Gauteng, South Africa: ARHAP, 2005.

African Religious Health Assets Programme (ARHAP). *ARHAP International Colloquium 2007: Monkey Valley Resort, Cape Town, South Africa, March 13–16, 2007, Collection of Concept Papers*.

Co-sponsored by Methodist Healthcare, University of Cape Town, Vesper Society, and Emory University. Cape Town: ARHAP, 2007.

African Religious Health Assets Programme. *Assessing and Mobilizing Religious Health Assets in Christian Settings: Interim Report on a Study Conducted by Difaem and WCC. When Religion and Health Align: Mobilizing Religious Health Assets for Transformation, ARHAP Conference, Cape Town, 13–16 July 2009*. Cape Town: ARHAP, 2009.

Agarwal, Sabrina C. and Bonnie A. Glencross, eds. *Social Bioarchaeology*. Malden, MA: Wiley-Blackwell, 2011.

Anderson, Gary. *Charity: The Place of the Poor in the Biblical Tradition*. New Haven: Yale University Press, 2013.

Amesbury, Richard and George M. Newlands. *Faith and Human Rights: Christianity and the Global Struggle for Human Dignity*. Minneapolis: Fortress, 2008.

Backman, Gunilla, Paul Hunt, Rajat Khosla, Camila Jaramillo-Strouss, Belachew Mekuria Fikre, Caroline Rumble, David Pevalin, David Acurio Páez, Mónica Armijos Pineda, Ariel Frisancho, Duniska Torco, Mitra Motlagh, Dana Farcasanu, and Cristian Vladescu. "Health Systems and the Right to Health: An Assessment of 194 Countries." *The Lancet* 372 (December 13, 2008): 2047–85.

Bagchi, S. C. and S. C. Banerjee. "The Kumbh Fair (1966): Aspects of Environmental Sanitation and Other Related Measures." *Indian Journal of Public Health* 11, no. 4 (1967): 180–84.

Baker, S. Josephine. *Fighting for Life*. New York: Macmillan Publishing Co., 1939, reprinted Huntington, NY: Robert E. Krieger Publishing Co. Inc., 1980.

Banchoff, Thomas and Robert Wuthnow, eds. *Religion and the Global Politics of Human Rights*. New York: Oxford University Press, 2011.

Banerjee, Abhijit V. and Esther Duflo. *Poor Economics: A Radical Rethinking of the Way to Fight Global Poverty*. New York: Public Affairs, 2011.

Banks, A. Leslie, "Religious Fairs and Festivals in India." *The Lancet* 277, no. 7169 (January 21, 1961): 162–63.

Barnett, Michael and Janice Gross Stein. *Sacred Aid: Faith and Humanitarianism*. New York: Oxford University Press, 2012.

Barnett, Michael. *Empire of Humanity: A History of Humanitarianism.* Ithaca: Cornell University Press, 2011.

Bartkowski, John P. and Helen A. Regis. *Charitable Choices: Religion, Race, and Poverty in the Post-Welfare Era.* New York: New York University Press, 2003.

Bartram, Jamie and Sandy Cairncross, "Hygiene, Sanitation, and Water: Forgotten Foundations of Health." *PLoS Medicine* 7, no. 11 (November 2010): e1000367.

Beetham, David. "What Future for Economic and Social Rights?" *Political Studies* 43 (1995): 41–60.

Belshaw, Deryke and Christopher Sugden, eds. *Faith in Development: Partnership Between the World Bank and the Churches of Africa.* Washington, DC: World Bank Publications, and Oxford: Regnum Books International, 2001.

Beracochea, Elvira, Corey Weinstein, and Dabney P. Evans, eds. *Rights-Based Approaches to Public Health.* New York: Springer Publishing Company, 2011.

Biéler, André. *Calvin's Economic and Social Thought.* Edited by Edward Dommen, translated by James Greig. Geneva: World Alliance of Reformed Churches and World Council of Churches, 2005.

Birn, Anne-Emanuelle and Theodore M. Brown, eds. *Comrades in Health: U.S. Health Internationalists, Abroad and at Home.* New Brunswick, NJ: Rutgers University Press, 2013.

Birn, Anne-Emanuelle, Yogan Pillay, and Timothy H. Holtz, eds. *Textbook of International Health: Global Health in a Dynamic World.* 3rd ed. New York: Oxford University Press, 2009.

Block, Jennie Weiss and Michael Griffin, eds. *In the Company of the Poor: Conversations with Dr. Paul Farmer and Fr. Gustavo Gutiérrez.* Maryknoll, NY: Orbis Books, 2013.

Bonner, Michael, Mine Ener, and Amy Singer, eds. *Poverty and Charity in Middle Eastern Contexts.* Albany: State University of New York Press, 2003.

Bos, Gerrit, trans. *Qusṭā ibn Lūqā al-Baʿlabakkī's Medical Regime for the Pilgrims to Mecca: The Risāla fī tadbīr safar al-hajj.* Islamic Philosophy, Theology and Science: Texts and Studies 11. Leiden: Brill, 1992.

Bradley, Elizabeth H. and Lauren A. Taylor. *The American Health Care Paradox: Why Spending More Is Getting Us Less*. New York: Public Affairs, 2013.

Bretherton, Luke. *Resurrecting Democracy: Faith, Citizenship and the Politics of a Common Life*. Cambridge Studies in Social Theory, Religion and Politics. New York: Cambridge University Press, 2014.

Bretherton, Luke. *Hospitality as Holiness: Christian Witness Amid Moral Diversity*. Aldershot: Ashgate, 2006.

Brodsky, Alyn. *Benjamin Rush: Patriot and Physician*. New York: St. Martin's Press, 2004.

Brown, Peter. *Through the Eye of a Needle: Wealth, the Fall of Rome, and the Making of Christianity in the West, 350–550 AD*. Princeton: Princeton University Press, 2012.

Brüning, Alfons and Evert van der Zweerde, eds. *Orthodox Christianity and Human Rights*. Eastern Christian Studies 13. Leuven: Peeters, 2012.

Bryceson, A. D. M. "Cholera, the Flickering Flame." *Proceedings of the Royal Society of Medicine* 70 (1977): 363–65.

Byrne, Patrick H. "Universal Rights or Personal Relations?" In *Christianity and Human Rights: Christians and the Struggle for Global Justice*, edited by Frederick M. Shepherd, 99–118. Lanham, MD: Lexington Books, 2009.

Cahill, Lisa Sowle. "Justice for Women: Martha Nussbaum and Catholic Social Teaching." In *Transforming Unjust Structures: The Capability Approach*, edited by Séverine Deneulin, Mathias Nebel, and Nicholas Sagovsky, 83–104. Library of Ethics and Applied Philosophy 19. Dordrecht, The Netherlands: Springer, 2006.

Caldwell, Melissa L. *Not by Bread Alone: Social Support in the New Russia*. Berkeley: University of California Press, 2004.

Campbell, Ted A. *John Wesley and Christian Antiquity: Religious Vision and Cultural Change*. Nashville: Kingswood Books, 1991.

Caner, Daniel F. "Alms, Blessings, Offerings: The Repertoire of Christian Gifts in Early Byzantium." In *The Gift in Antiquity*, edited by Michael Satlow, 25–44. The Ancient World: Comparative Histories. Malden, MA: Wiley-Blackwell, 2013.

Capasso, Luigi and Luisa Di Domenicantonio. "Work-Related Syndesmoses on the Bones of Children Who Died at Herculaneum" [Letter]. *The Lancet* 352, no. 9140 (1998): 1634.

Capasso, Luigi. "Indoor Pollution and Respiratory Diseases in Ancient Rome" [letter]. *The Lancet* 356 (2000): 1774.

Caputo, John D. and Michael J. Scanlon, eds. *God, The Gift, and Postmodernism*. Bloomington, IN: Indiana University Press, 1999.

Carey, Matthew. *Essays on the Public Charities of Philadelphia, Intended to Vindicate the Benevolent Societies of this City from the Charge of Encouraging Idleness, and to Place in Strong Relief, before an Enlightened Public, the Sufferings and Oppression under which the Greater Part of the Females Labour, Who Depend on Their Industry for a Support for Themselves and Children*. 4th ed. Philadelphia: J. Clarke, 1829.

Castro, Arachu and Merrill Singer, eds. *Unhealthy Health Policy: A Critical Anthropological Examination*. Lanham, MD: Altamira Press, 2004.

Center for Human Rights and Global Justice (CHRGJ), RFK Center for Justice and Human Rights, Partners In Health, and Zanmi Lasante. *Wòch Nan Soley: The Denial of the Right to Water in Haiti*. 2008.

Center for Human Rights and Global Justice (CHRGJ), RFK Center for Justice and Human Rights, Partners In Health, and Zanmi Lasante. *Sak Vid Pa Kanpe: The Impact of US Food Aid on Human Rights in Haiti*. 2010.

Cheah, Elena. *An Orchestra Beyond Borders: Voices of the West-Eastern Divan Orchestra*. London: Verso, 2009.

Chilton, M., M. M. Black, C. Berkowitz, P. H. Casey, J. Cook, D. Cutts, R. R. Jacobs, T. Heeren, S. Ettinger de Cuba, S. Coleman, A. Meyers, and D. A. Franks. "Food Insecurity and Risk of Poor Health among US-Born Children of Immigrants. *American Journal of Public Health* 99, no. 3 (2009): 556–62.

Clooney, Francis X. *Comparative Theology: Deep Learning Across Religious Borders*. Malden, MA: Wiley-Blackwell, 2010.

Cochrane, James R. "Agapé: The Cape Office of the Christian Institute." *Journal of Theology for Southern Africa* 118 (March 2004): 53–68.

Cochrane, James R. "Being Accountable for the Life of Religious Health Assets." Keynote Address, *Christian Responses to Global Health and Development*, International Symposium 50 Years after 'Tübingen I,' Deutsches Institute für ärzliche Mission (Difäm). Tübingen, Germany, June 26–29, 2014.

Cochrane, James R. *Circles of Dignity: Community Wisdom and Theological Reflection*. Minneapolis: Fortress Press, 1999.

Cochrane, James R. "Fire from Above, Fire from Below: Health, Justice and the Persistence of the Sacred." *Theoria* 55, no. 116 (August 2008): 67–96.

Cochrane, James R. "Religion in the Health of Migrant Communities: Asset or Deficit?" *Journal of Ethnic and Migration Studies* 32, no. 4 (May 2006): 715–36.

Cochrane, James R. "Religion, Public Health and a Church for the 21st Century." *International Review of Mission* 95, nos. 376–77 (January 2006): 59–72.

Cochrane, James R. "The Language that Difference Makes." *Practical Matters* 4 (Spring 2011): 1–16.

Cochrane, James R. and Gary R. Gunderson. *The Barefoot Guide to Mobilizing Religious Health Assets for Transformation*. The Third Barefoot Collective. November 2012. http://www.barefootguide.org/barefoot-guide-3.html.

Cochrane, James R., Barbara Schmid, and Teresa Cutts, eds. *When Religion and Health Align: Mobilizing Religious Health Assets for Transformation*. Dorpspruit, South Africa: Cluster Publications, 2011.

Cochrane, James R., Elias Bongmba, Isabel Phiri, and Des van der Water. *Living on the Edge: Essays in Honour of Steve de Gruchy, Activist and Theologian*. Pietermaritzburg, South Africa: Cluster Publications, 2012.

Cole, Charles Chester. *Lion of the Forest: James B. Finley, Frontier Reformer*. Lexington, KY: University Press of Kentucky, 1994.

Collins, Daryl, Jonathan Murduch, Stuart Rutherford, and Orlanda Ruthven. *Portfolios of the Poor: How the World's Poor Live on $2 a Day*. Princeton, NJ: Princeton University Press, 2009.

Commission on Social Determinants of Health. *Closing the Gap in a Generation: Health Equity Through Action on the Social Determinants of Health Commission on Social Determinants of Health Final Report*. Geneva: World Health Organization, 2008.

Constantelos, Demetrios J. *Byzantine Philanthropy and Social Welfare*. 2nd edition. New Rochelle, NY: A. D. Caratzas, 1991.

Constanzo, Eric. *Harbor for the Poor: A Missiological Analysis of Almsgiving in the View and Practice of John Chrysostom*. Eugene, OR: Pickwick Publications, 2013.

Corbett, Steve and Brian Fikkert. *When Helping Hurts: How to Alleviate Poverty without Hurting the Poor and Yourself*. Chicago: Moody Publishers, 2009.

Courtney, Jennifer. *Keeping Faith: Faith Responses to HIV and AIDS: Mapping the Future*. London: UK Consortium on AIDS and International Development, 2011.

Crislip, Andrew. *From Monastery to Hospital: Christian Monasticism and the Transformation of Health Care in Antiquity*. Grand Rapids: University of Michigan Press, 2005.

Crislip, Andrew. *Thorns in the Flesh: Illness and Sanctity in Late Antique Christianity*. Divinations: Rereading Late Ancient Religion; Philadelphia: University of Pennsylvania Press, 2012.

Cutts T. "The Memphis Congregational Health Network model: grounding ARHAP theory." In *When Religion and Health Align: Mobilizing Religious Health Assets for Transformation*, edited by B. Schmid, J. R. Cochrane, and T. Cutts, 193–209. Pietermaritzburg, South Africa: Cluster Publications, 2011.

Cutts, Teresa F., Gary R. Gunderson, Rae Jean Proeschold-Bell, and Robin Swift. "The life of leaders: An intensive health program for clergy." *Journal of Religious Health* 51 (2012): 1317–24.

Danaher, Kevin, ed. *50 Years Is Enough: The Case Against the World Bank and the International Monetary Fund*. Boston: South End Press, 1999.

Daniels, Margarette. *Makers of South America*. New York: Missionary Education Movement of the US and Canada, 1916.

Davey, Francis. *Richard of Lincoln: A Medieval Doctor Travels to Jerusalem*. Exeter, UK: Azure Publications, 2013.

De Gruchy, John W. with Steve de Gruchy. *The Church Struggle in South Africa, 25th Anniversary Edition*. Minneapolis: Fortress Press, 2005.

De Gruchy, Steve, "Of Agency, Assets and Appreciation: Seeking Some Commonalities between Theology and Development." *Journal of Theology for Southern Africa* 117 (November 2003): 20–39.

De Gruchy, Steve, Nico Koopman, and Sytse Strijbos, eds. *From Our Side: Emerging Perspectives on Development and Ethics*.

Amsterdam, The Netherlands: Rozenberg Publishers/West Lafayette, Indiana: Purdue University Press, 2008.

De Gruchy, Steve. "Dealing with Our Own Sewage: Spirituality and Ethics in the Sustainability Agenda: Address to the World Conference on Theologies of Liberation, Belem, Brazil, January 2009." *Journal of Theology for Southern Africa* 134 (2009): 53–65.

De Gruchy, Steve. "Water and the Spirit: Theology in the Time of Cholera." *World Council of Churches Ecumenical Review* 62, no. 2 (July 2010): 188–201.

Deneulin, Séverine and Carole Rakodi. "Revisiting Religion: Development Studies Thirty Years On." *World Development* 39, no. 1 (2011): 45–54. doi:10.1016/j.worlddev.2010.05.007.

Deneulin, Séverine. "Development and the Limits of Amartya Sen's *The Idea of Justice*." *Third World Quarterly* 32, no. 4 (2011): 787–97.

Deneulin, Séverine. *Wellbeing, Justice and Development Ethics.* The Routledge Human Development and Capability Debates. New York: Routledge, 2014.

Dix, Dorothea. *Remarks on Prisons and Prison Discipline in the United States.* Boston: Munroe & Francis, 1845.

Doran, Robert, trans. *Stewards of the Poor: The Man of God, Rabbula, and Hiba in Fifth-Century Edessa.* Cistercian Studies Series 208. Kalamazoo, MI: Cistercian Publications, 2006.

Doran, Robert, trans. *The Lives of Simeon Stylites.* Cistercian Studies Series 112. Kalamazoo, MI: Cistercian Publications, 1992.

Eck, Diana. *Darśan: Seeing the Divine Image in India.* 3rd ed. New York: Columbia University Press, 1998.

Elliott, Samuel Hayes. *New England's Chattels: or, Life in the Northern Poor House.* New York: H. Dayton, 1858.

Elm, Susanna. "Developments in Ancient Medicine: Models for Today's Challenges?" In: *Medical Challenges for the New Millennium: An Interdisciplinary Task,* edited by Stefan N. Willich and Susanna Elm, 3–20. Dordrecht, The Netherlands: Kluwer Academic Publishers, 2001.

Ely, Ezra Stiles. *A Sermon for the Rich to Buy that They May Benefit Themselves and the Poor.* New York: Williams and Whiting, 1810.

Ely, Ezra Stiles. *The Second Journal of the Stated Preacher to the Hospital and Almshouse in the City of New York for a Part of the Year of Our Lord 1813.* Philadelphia: M. Cary, 1815.

Emmons, Robert A. and Michael E. McCullough, eds. *The Psychology of Gratitude*. New York: Oxford University Press, 2004.

Fa-Hsien. *The Travels of Fa-hsien (399–414 A.D.), or Record of the Buddhistic Kingdoms*. Translated by H. A. Giles. New York: Cambridge University Press, 1923, reprinted 2011.

Farmer, Paul. *Haiti After the Earthquake*. Edited by Abbey Gardner and Cassia Van Der Hoof Holstein. New York: Public Affairs, 2011.

Farmer, Paul. *Partner to the Poor: A Paul Farmer Reader*. Edited by Haun Saussay. Berkeley: University of California Press, 2010.

Farmer, Paul. *Pathologies of Power: Health, Human Rights, and the New War on the Poor*. Berkeley: University of California Press, 2005.

Farmer, Paul. *To Repair the World: Paul Farmer Speaks to the Next Generation*. Edited by Jonathan Weigel. Berkeley: University of California Press, 2013.

Farmer, Paul, Jim Yong Kim, Arthur Kleinman, and Matthew Basilico, eds. *Reimagining Global Health: An Introduction*. Berkeley: University of California Press, 2013.

Farmer, Sharon. *Surviving Poverty in Medieval Paris: Gender, Ideology, and the Daily Lives of the Poor*. Ithaca, NY: Cornell University Press, 2002.

Finley, James Bradley. *Memorials of Prison Life*. Edited by Rev. B. F. Tefft. Cincinnati: L. Swormstedt & A. Poe, 1853.

Food and Agriculture Organization (FAO), World Food Programme (WFP), and International Fund for Agricultural Development (IFAD). *The State of Food Insecurity in the World 2012: Economic Growth Is Necessary but Not Sufficient to Accelerate Reduction of Hunger and Malnutrition*. Rome: FAO, 2012.

Fortman, Bas de Gaay and Berma Klein Goldewijk. *God and the Goods: Global Economy in a Civilizational Perspective*. Geneva: World Council of Churches, 1998.

Fortman, Bas de Gaay. *Political Economy of Human Rights: Rights, Realities and Realization*. Routledge Frontiers of Political Economy. London: Routledge, 2011.

Fortman, Bas de Gaay and Jacques Paul Klein. *Peace in the 21st Century: Between the Supranational and the Grassroots*. Wageningen, the Netherlands: Educatief Centrum 'Hotel De Wereld,' 2000.

Foster, Geoff, comp. *Study of the Response by Faith-Based Organizations to Orphans and Vulnerable Children: Preliminary Summary Report.* World Conference of Religions for Peace. New York: UNICEF, 2004.

Foster, Geoff. "HIV/AIDS Policy Initiatives: Learning from Christian Involvement in Health Provision and Child Welfare Reform." *Journal of Family and Community Ministries* 24 (2009): 8–19.

Frank, Georgia. *The Memory of the Eyes: Pilgrims to Living Saints in Christian Late Antiquity.* Transformation of the Classical Heritage, 30. Berkeley: University of California Press, 2000.

Gardner, Gregg E. "Charity Wounds: Gifts to the Poor in Early Rabbinic Judaism." In *The Gift in Antiquity,* edited by Michael Satlow, 173–88. The Ancient World: Comparative Histories. Malden, MA: Wiley-Blackwell, 2013.

Germond, Paul and James R. Cochrane. "Healthworlds: Conceptualizing Landscapes of Health and Healing." *Sociology* 44 (2010): 307–24; doi: 10.1177/0038038509357202.

Gilson, Lucy. "The Relevance of Healthworlds to Health System Thinking about Access." In *When Religion and Health Align Mobilizing Religious Health Assets for Transformation,* edited by James R. Cochrane, Barbara Schmid, and Teresa Cutts, 164–77. Dorpspruit, South Africa: Cluster Publications, 2011.

Glendon, Mary Ann. *A World Made New: Eleanor Roosevelt and the Universal Declaration of Human Rights.* New York: Random House, 2001.

Global Fund to Fight AIDS, Tuberculosis, and Malaria. *Report on the Involvement of Faith-Based Organizations in the Global Fund,* 2008, 2010 update. http://www.theglobalfund.org/en/civilsociety/reports/.

Goizueta, Roberto S. *Caminemos con Jesús: Toward a Hispanic/Latino Theology of Accompaniment.* Maryknoll, NY: Orbis Books, 1995.

Goldewijk, Berma Klein and Bas de Gaay Fortman. *Where Needs Meet Rights: Economic, Social and Cultural Rights in a New Perspective.* Geneva: World Council of Churches, 1999.

Goodman, Amy and Denis Moynihan. *The Silenced Majority: Stories of Uprisings, Occupations, Resistance, and Hope.* Chicago: Haymarket Books, 2012.

Goodpasture, H. McKennie. "David Trumbull: Missionary Journalist and Liberty in Chile, 1845–1889." *Journal of Presbyterian History* 56, no. 2 (1978): 149–65.

Gornik, Mark R. *Word Made Global: Stories of African Christianity in New York City.* Grand Rapids: Eerdmans, 2011.

Gornik, Mark R. *To Live in Peace: Biblical Faith and the Changing Inner City.* Grand Rapids: Eerdmans, 2002.

Gray, Alyssa M. "The Formerly Wealthy Poor: From Empathy to Ambivalence in Rabbinic Literature of Late Antiquity." *AJS Review* 33, no. 1 (2009): 101–33; doi: 10.1017/S0364009409000051.

Gregory, Eric. "Agape and Special Relations in a Global Economy: Theological Sources." In *Global Neighbors: Christian Faith and Moral Obligations in Today's Economy,* edited by Douglas A. Hicks and Mark Valeri, 16–41. Grand Rapids: Wm. B. Eerdmans, 2008.

Groody, Daniel G. *Globalization, Spirituality, and Justice.* Maryknoll, NY: Orbis, 2007.

Gunderson, Gary. *Boundary Leaders: Leadership Skills for People of Faith.* Minneapolis: Fortress Press, 2004.

Gunderson, Gary with Larry Pray. *Leading Causes of Life: Five Fundamentals to Change the Way You Live Your Life.* Nashville: Abingdon Press, 2009.

Gunderson, Gary R. "The other side of complexity: Faith, health, and humility" [Policy Forum]. *Virtual Mentor: Ethics Journal of the American Medical Association* 7, no. 5 (May 2005). http://virtual-mentor.ama-assn.org/2005/05/pdf/pfor1-0505.pdf.

Gunderson, Gary R. and James R. Cochrane. *Religion and the Health of the Public: Shifting the Paradigm.* New York: Palgrave Macmillan, 2012.

Haddad, Beverley, Jill Olivier, and Steve de Gruchy. *The Potentials and Perils of Partnership: Christian Religious Entities and Collaborative Stakeholders Responding to HIV in Kenya, Malawi and the DRC: Summary Report.* Study commissioned by Tearfund and UNAIDS. Cape Town: ARHAP 2009.

Halperin, Alex. "It Really Does Take a Village: How Memphis is Fixing Healthcare." *Salon.com,* September 3, 2013. http://www.salon.com/2013/09/03/it_really_does_take_a_village_how_memphis_is_fixing_healthcare/.

Hannum, Hurst. "The Status of the Universal Declaration of Human Rights in National and International Law." *Georgia Journal of International and Comparative Law*, 25, nos. 1–2 (1995/1996): 287–397.

Harper, Kyle. *Slavery in the Late Roman World AD 275–425.* New York: Cambridge University Press, 2011.

Hartman, Laura M. *The Christian Consumer: Living Faithfully in a Fragile World.* New York: Oxford University Press, 2011.

Hénaff, Marcel. *The Price of Truth: Gift, Money, and Philosophy.* Trans. Jean-Louis Morhange with the collaboration of Anne-Marie Feenberg-Dibon. Stanford: Stanford University Press, 2010.

Herbert, H. "The Natural History of Hardwar Fair Cholera Outbreaks." *The Lancet* 146, no. 3752 (July 27, 1895): 201–02.

Hicks, Donna. *Dignity: The Essential Role It Plays in Resolving Conflict.* New Haven: Yale University Press, 2011.

Holman, Susan R. *God Knows There's Need: Christian Responses to Poverty.* New York: Oxford University Press, 2009.

Holman, Susan R. "Healing the World with Righteousness? The Language of Social Justice in Early Christian Homilies." In *Charity and Giving in Monotheistic Religions,* edited by Miriam Frenkel and Yaacov Lev, 89–110. Studien zur Geschichte und Kultur des islamischen Orients. Berlin: De Gruyter, 2009.

Holman, Susan R. "Martyr-Saints and the Demon of Infant Mortality: Folk Healing in Early Christian Pediatric Medicine." In *Children and Family in Late Antiquity: Life, Death and Interaction,* edited by Christian Laes, Katariina Mustakallio, and Ville Vuolanto, 233–54. Interdisciplinary Studies in Ancient Culture and Religion 15; Leuven: Peeters, 2014.

Holman, Susan R. "On the Ground: Realizing an 'Altared' Philoptochia." In *Philanthropy and Social Compassion in Eastern Orthodox Tradition,* edited by Matthew Pereira, 31–49. Papers of the Sophia Institute Annual Academic Conference Dec. 2009. New York: Theotokos Press, 2010.

Holman, Susan R. "Out of the Fitting Room: Rethinking Patristic Social Texts on 'The Common Good.'" In *Reading Patristic Texts on Social Ethics: Issues and Challenges for 21st-Century Christian Social Thought,* edited by Johan Leemans, Brian Matz, and Johan

Verstraeten, 103–23. Washington: Catholic University of America Press, 2011.

Holman, Susan R. "Sick Children and Healing Saints: Medical Treatment of the Child in Christian Antiquity." In *Children in Late Ancient Christianity*, edited by Cornelia B. Horn and Robert R. Phenix, 143–70. Studien und Texte zum Antiken Christentum/Studies and Texts on Ancient Christianity; Tübingen: Mohr-Siebeck, 2009.

Holman, Susan R. *The Hungry Are Dying: Beggars and Bishops in Roman Cappadocia.* New York: Oxford University Press, 2001.

Holman, Susan R. and Mark DelCogliano, trans. *St. Basil the Great on Fasting and Feasts.* Popular Patristics Series 50. Yonkers, NY: St. Vladimir Seminary Press, 2013.

Holman, Susan R. ed., *Wealth and Poverty in Early Church and Society.* Holy Cross Studies in Patristic Theology and History. Grand Rapids, MI: BakerAcademic/Holy Cross Greek Orthodox Press, 2008.

Huber, Wolfgang. "Human Rights and Globalisation: Are Human Rights a 'Western' Concept or a Universalistic Principle?" *Nederduitse Gereformeerde Teologiese Tydskrif (NGTT DEEL)* 55, no. 1 (2014): 117–137.

Hulme, Kathryn. *The Wild Place.* Boston: Little Brown, 1953.

Humphrey, John P. *Human Rights and the United Nations: A Great Adventure.* Dobbs Ferry, NY: Transnational Publishers, 1984.

Humphrey, John P. *On the Edge of Greatness: The Diaries of John Humphrey, First Director of the United Nations Division of Human Rights. Volume 1, 1948–1949.* Edited by A. J. Hobbins. Fontanus Monograph Series 4. Montreal: McGill University Libraries, 1994.

Idler, Ellen L., ed. *Religion as a Social Determinant of Public Health: Interdisciplinary Inquiries.* New York: Oxford University Press, 2014.

Ignatieff, Michael. *Human Rights as Politics and Idolatry.* Edited by Amy Gutmann. Princeton: Princeton University Press, 2001.

Ignatieff, Michael. *The Needs of Strangers.* New York: Picador USA, 1984.

Ihssen, Brenda Llewellyn. *They Who Give from Evil: The Response of the Eastern Church to Moneylending in the Early Christian Era.* Eugene, OR: Wipf and Stock, 2012.

Ishay, Micheline R. *The History of Human Rights: From Ancient Times to the Globalization Era.* Berkeley: University of California Press, 2004.

Jackson, Michael. *Life Within Limits: Well-Being in a World of Want.* Durham, NC: Duke University Press, 2011.

Jennings, Theodore W., Jr. *Good News to the Poor: John Wesley's Evangelical Economics.* Nashville: Abingdon, 1990.

Johnson, Steven. *The Ghost Map: The Story of London's Most Terrifying Epidemic—and How It Changed Science, Cities, and the Modern World.* New York: Riverhead Books, 2006.

Kagawa, Rose Calnin, Andrew Anglemyer, and Dominic Montagu. "The Scale of Faith-Based Organization Participation in Health Service Delivery in Developing Countries: Systematic Review and Meta-Analysis." *PLoS One* 7, no. 11 (November 2012), doi: e48457.

Karpf, Ted and Alex Ross, eds. *Building from Common Foundations: The World Health Organization and Faith-Based Organizations in Primary Healthcare.* Geneva: Geneva Global Performance Philanthropy and the World Health Organization, 2008.

Karpf, Ted, J. Todd Ferguson, Robin Swift, and Jeffrey V. Lazarus, eds. *Restoring Hope: Decent Care in the midst of HIV/AIDS.* New York: Palgrave Macmillan, 2008.

Katz, Michael B. *In the Shadow of the Poorhouse: A Social History of Welfare in America.* New York: Basic Books, 1986.

Kemble, John Haskell. *The Panama Route 1848–1869.* Columbus, SC: University of South Carolina Press, 1990.

Kemp, Barry, Anna Stevens, Gretchen R. Dabbs, Melissa Zabecki, and Jerome C. Rose. "Life, Death and Beyond in Akhenaton's Egypt: Excavating the South Tombs Cemetery at Amarna." *Antiquity* 87 (2013): 64–78.

Kiser, Miriam, Deborah L. Jones, and Gary R. Gunderson. "Faith and Health: Leadership Aligning Assets to Transform Communities." *International Review of Mission* vol. 95, nos. 376–77 (January/April 2006), 50–58.

Knighton-Fitt, Jean. *Beyond Fear: In South Africa's Darkest Days—Theo and Helen Kotze: A Sign to the World on Turning Injustice and Hurt into a Celebration of Friendship.* Cape Town: PreText Publishers, 2003.

Knudsen, Milli S. *Hard Times in Concord, New Hampshire: The Crimes, the Victims, and the Lives of State Prison Inmates 1812–1883.* Westminster, MD: Heritage Books, 2008.

Komter, Aafke E. *Social Solidarity and the Gift.* New York: Cambridge University Press, 2005.

Kretzman, John P. and John L. McKnight. *Building Communities from the Inside Out: A Path Toward Finding and Mobilizing a Community's Assets.* Chicago: ACTA Publications. 1993.

Küng, Hans and Helmut Schmidt, eds. *A Global Ethic and Global Responsibility: Two Declarations.* London: SCM Press, 1998.

Lactantius. *Lactantius: Divine Institutes.* Edited and translated by Anthony Bowen and Peter Garnsey. Translated Texts for Historians. Liverpool, UK: Liverpool University Press, 2004.

Laksana, A. Bagus. "Comparative Theology: Between Identity and Alterity." In *The New Comparative Theology: Interreligious Insights from the Next Generation,* edited by Francis X. Clooney, 1–20. London: T&T Clark, 2010.

Leemans, Johan, Brian Matz, and Johan Verstraeten, eds. *Reading Patristic Texts on Social Ethics: Issues and Challenges for 21st-Century Christian Social Thought.* Washington: Catholic University of America Press, 2011.

LeVine, Robert A., Sarah LeVine, Beatrice Schnell-Anzola, Meredith L. Rowe, and Emily Dexter. *Literacy and Mothering: How Women's Schooling Changes the Lives of the World's Children.* New York: Oxford University Press, 2012.

Levine, Ruth and the What Works Working Group, with Molly Kinder. *Case Studies in Global Health: Millions Saved.* Burlington MA: Jones and Bartlett, 2007.

Levinson, Justin D. and Robert J. Smith, eds. *Implicit Racial Bias Across the Law.* New York: Cambridge University Press, 2012.

Lindberg, Carter. *Beyond Charity: Reformation Initiatives for the Poor.* Minneapolis: Fortress, 1993.

Longenecker, Bruce W. and Kelly D. Liebengood, eds. *Engaging Economics: New Testament Scenarios and Early Christian Reception.* Grand Rapids: Eerdmans, 2009.

Longenecker, Bruce. *Remember the Poor: Paul, the Poor and the Graeco-Roman World.* Grand Rapids: Eerdmans, 2010.

López, Ariel. *Shenoute of Atripe and the Uses of Poverty: Rural Patronage, Religious Conflict, and Monasticism in Late Antique Egypt.* Berkeley: University of California Press, 2013.

Loy, David R. "The Poverty of Development: Buddhist Reflections." *Development* 46, no. 4 (2003): 7–14.

Lumbard, Joseph. "Some Reflections on Hospitality in Islam." In *Hosting the Stranger: Between Religions,* edited by Richard Kearney and James Taylor, 133–38. New York: Continuum, 2011.

MacIntyre, Alasdair. *After Virtue.* Notre Dame, IN: University of Notre Dame Press, 1981.

Maclean, Kama. *Pilgrimage and Power: The Kumbh Mela in Allahabad, 1765–1954.* New York: Oxford University Press, 2008.

MacMillan, Malcolm. *An Odd Kind of Fame: Stories of Phineas Gage.* Cambridge: MIT Press, 2002.

Mann, Jonathan M., Sofia Gruskin, Michael A. Grodin, and George J. Annas, eds. *Health and Human Rights: A Reader.* New York: Routledge, 1999.

Maren, Michael. *The Road to Hell: The Ravaging Effects of Foreign Aid and International Charity.* New York: The Free Press, 1997.

Marion, Jean-Luc. *Being Given: Toward a Phenomenology of Givenness,* translated by Jeffrey L. Kosky. Stanford: Stanford University Press, 2002.

Maritain, Jacques. *Scholasticism and Politics.* New York: The MacMillan Co., 1940.

Marks, Stephen P. "The Past and Future of the Separation of Human Rights into Categories." *Maryland Journal of International Law* 24 (2009): 209–43.

Marmot, Michael and Richard G. Wilkinson, eds. *Social Determinants of Health.* 2nd ed. New York: Oxford University Press, 2005.

Marshall, Katherine. "A Discussion with Reverend Canon Ted Karpf." Berkley Center for Religion, Peace & World Affairs, Georgetown University, November 13, 2010. http://berkleycenter.georgetown. edu/interviews/a-discussion-with-reverend-canon-ted-karpf.

Marshall, Katherine. *Global Institutions of Religion: Ancient Movers, Modern Shakers.* Routledge Global Institutions Series. New York: Routledge, 2013.

Mash, Rachel and Robert Mash. "Faith-Based Organizations and HIV Prevention in Africa: A Review." *African Journal of Primary Health Care Family Medicine* 5, no. 1 (2013). http://dx.doi.org/10.4102/phcfm.v5i1.464.

Mathai, Rabia for JLICA Learning Group 2. *The Role of Faith-Based Organizations (FBOs) in Providing Care and Support to Children Living with and Affected by HIV and AIDS and FBO Collaboration with and Integration within National HIV Responses.* Boston: JLICA, 2009.

Mathewes, Charles. *A Theology of Public Life.* New York: Cambridge University Press, 2007.

Mauss, Marcel. *The Gift: The Form and Reason for Exchange in Archaic Societies.* Edited by W. D. Hall, with a foreword by Mary Douglas. New York: W. W. Norton, 1990.

Memish, Ziad A., Gwen M. Stephens, Robert Steffen, and Qanta A. Ahmed. "Emergence of Medicine for Mass Gatherings: Lessons from the Hajj." *The Lancet Infectious Diseases* 12, no.1 (2012): 56–65.

Miller, Patricia Cox. *The Corporeal Imagination: Signifying the Holy in Late Ancient Christianity.* Divinations: Rereading Late Ancient Religion. Philadelphia: University of Pennsylvania Press, 2009.

Miller, Timothy S. *The Birth of the Hospital in the Byzantine Empire.* Baltimore: Johns Hopkins Press, 1997.

Morgan, David. *The Sacred Gaze: Religious Visual Culture in Theory and Practice.* Berkeley: University of California Press, 2005.

Morsink, Johannes. *Inherent Human Rights: Philosophical Roots of the Universal Declaration.* Philadelphia: University of Pennsylvania Press, 2009.

Morsink, Johannes. *The Universal Declaration of Human Rights: Origins, Drafting and Intent.* Philadelphia: University of Pennsylvania Press, 1999.

Moyn, Samuel. *The Last Utopia: Human Rights in History.* Cambridge, MA: Harvard University Press, 2010.

Moyo, Dambisa. *Dead Aid: Why Aid Is Not Working and How There Is a Better Way for Africa.* New York: Farrar, Straus and Giroux, 2010.

Murdock, Carl J. "Physicians, the State and Public Health in Chile, 1881–1891." *Journal of Latin American Studies* 27, no. 3 (1995): 551–67.

Murthy, Sharmila L. "The Human Right(s) to Water and Sanitation: History, Meaning and the Controversy Over Privatization." *Berkeley Journal of International Law* 31, no. 1 (2013): 89–149.

Myers, Bryant. *Walking with the Poor: Principles and Practices of Transformational Development.* Revised edition. Maryknoll, NY: Orbis, 2011.

Narayan, Deepa and Patti Patesch, eds. *Voices of the Poor: From Many Lands.* [vol. 3.] Washington, DC, and New York: Oxford University Press for the World Bank, 2002.

Narayan, Deepa with Raj Patel, Kai Schafft, Anne Rademacher, and Sarah Koch-Schulte, eds. *Voices of the Poor: Can Anyone Hear Us?* [vol. 1.] Washington, DC, and New York: Oxford University Press for the World Bank, 2000.

Narayan, Deepa, Robert Chambers, Meera Kaul Shah, Patti Petesch, eds. *Voices of the Poor: Crying out for Change.* [vol. 2.] Washington, DC, and New York: Oxford University Press for the World Bank, 2000.

Navarro, Vicente. "What we mean by Social Determinants of Health." *International Journal of Health Services* 39, no. 3 (2009): 423–41.

Nurser, John. *For All People and All Nations: Christian Churches and Human Rights.* Geneva: World Council of Churches Publications, 2005.

Novick, Tzvi. "Charity and Reciprocity: Structures of Benevolence in Rabbinic Literature." *Harvard Theological Review* 105, no. 1 (2012): 33–52.

Nussbaum, Martha C. "Equity and Mercy." *Philosophy and Public Affairs* 22 (1993): 83–125.

Nussbaum, Martha C. *Creating Capabilities: The Human Development Approach.* Cambridge, MA: Harvard University Press, 2011.

Olivier, Jill and Quentin Wodon, eds. *Strengthening the Evidence for Faith-Inspired Health Engagement in Africa.* 3 vols. HNP Discussion Paper Series. Washington, DC: The World Bank, 2012.

Olivier, Jill, James R. Cochrane, and Barbara Schmid, with Lauren Graham. *ARHAP Bibliography: Working in a Bounded Field of Unknowing.* Cape Town, South Africa: ARHAP, 2006.

Olivier, Jill, James R. Cochrane, and Barbara Schmid, with Lauren Graham. *ARHAP Literature Review: Working in a Bounded Field of Unknowing.* Cape Town, South Africa: ARHAP, 2006.

Olivier, Jill. "An FB-oh? Mapping the Etymologies of the Religious Entity Engaged in Health." In *When Religion and Health Align: Mobilizing Religious Health Assets for Transformation,* edited by James R. Cochrane, Barbara Schmid, and Teresa Cutts, 24–42. Pietermaritzburg, South Africa: Cluster Publications, 2011.

Osiek, Carolyn. *Rich and Poor in the Shepherd of Hermas: An Exegetical-Social Investigation.* The Catholic Biblical Quarterly Monograph Series 15. Washington, DC: The Catholic Biblical Association of America, 1983.

Partners In Health. *Program Management Guide.* Boston: Partners In Health, 2011. http://www.pih.org/library/pih-program-management-guide.

Pascale, Richard, Jerry Sternin, and Monique Sternin. *The Power of Positive Deviance: How Unlikely Innovators Solve the World's Toughest Problems.* Cambridge, MA: Harvard Business Review Press, 2010.

Paul, Irven. *A Yankee Reformer in Chile: The Life and Works of David Trumbull.* South Pasadena, CA: William Carey Library, 1973.

Perlman, Daniel and Ananya Roy. *The Practice of International Health: A Case-Based Orientation.* New York: Oxford University Press, 2009.

Pierre, Paul. "Moral Responsibility in a Context of Scarcity: The Journey of a Haitian Physician." *Narrative Inquiry in Bioethics* 2, no. 2 (Fall 2012): 89–92.

Pogge, Thomas. "Severe Poverty as a Violation of Negative Duties." *Ethics and International Affairs* 19, no. 1 (2005): 55–84.

Pogge, Thomas. *World Poverty and Human Rights.* 2nd ed. Cambridge, UK, and Malden, MA: Polity Press, 2008.

Pogrund, Benjamin. *How Can Man Die Better . . . Sobukwe and Apartheid.* London: Peter Halben, 1990.

Polman, Linda. *Crisis Caravan: What's Wrong with Humanitarian Aid?* Translated by Liz Waters. New York: Metropolitan Books, 2010.

Priestley, James. *A Charity Sermon Delivered in the Methodist Chapel, Halifax (Nova Scotia) on the Evening of Christmas Day.* Halifax: A. H. Holland, 1818.

Probasco, LiErin. "More Good than Harm: Moral Action and Evaluation in International Religious Volunteer Tourism." PhD Diss. Princeton University, 2013.

Prowse, Tracy L. "Diet and Dental Health Through the Life Course in Roman Italy." In *Social Bioarchaeology*, edited by Sabrina C. Agarwal and Bonnie A. Glencross, 410–37. Malden, MA: Wiley-Blackwell, 2011.

Prowse, T. L. "Isotopic and Dental Evidence for Infant and Young Child Feeding Practices in an Imperial Roman Skeletal Sample." *American Journal of Physical Anthropology* 137 (2008): 294–308.

Rasanathan, Kumanan for the World Health Organization. *Closing the Gap: Policy into Practice on Social Determinants of Health: Discussion Paper.* Rio de Janeiro: World Conference on Social Determinants of Health, October 19–21, 2011. http://www. who.int/sdhconference/Discussion-Paper-EN.pdf.

Reed, Esther D. *The Ethics of Human Rights: Contested Doctrinal and Moral Issues.* Waco, TX: Baylor University Press, 2007.

Regan, Ethna. *Theology and the Boundary Discourse of Human Rights.* Washington, DC: Georgetown University Press, 2010.

Reinikka, Ritva and Jakob Svensson. *Working for God? Evaluating Service Delivery of Religious Not-for-Profit Health Care Providers in Uganda.* Policy Research Working Paper 3058. Washington, DC: The World Bank Development Research Group, 2003.

Rhee, Helen. *Loving the Poor, Saving the Rich: Wealth, Poverty, and Early Christian Formation.* Grand Rapids: BakerAcademic, 2012.

Risse, Guenter B. *Mending Bodies, Saving Souls: A History of Hospitals.* New York: Oxford University Press, 1999.

Roberts, Joel. *The Cholera of 1849, and the Opinions of Medical and Other Professional Gentlemen, in Regards to Its Origin and Proper Treatment, Embracing the Alopathy, Homoeopathy, Electrical and Eclectic Theories and Prescriptions, Selected from the Various Journals of the Day.* Sandusky City, OH: W. S. Mills and Co., 1850.

Rosenberg, Charles E. *The Care of Strangers: The Rise of America's Hospital System.* New York: Basic Books, 1987.

Rosenberg, Charles E. *The Cholera Years: The United States in 1832, 1849, and 1866.* 2nd edition. Chicago: University of Chicago Press, 1987.

Rothman, Sheila M. *Living in the Shadow of Death: Tuberculosis and the Social Experience of Illness in American History.* Baltimore: Johns Hopkins University Press, 1994.

Ruger, Jennifer Prah. *Health and Social Justice.* New York: Oxford University Press, 2010.

Rush, Benjamin. *Medical Inquiries and Observations.* 3rd ed. 4 vols. Philadelphia: Matthew Carey, 1809.

Rush, David. "The National WIC Evaluation: Evaluation of the Special Supplemental Food Program for Women, Infants, and Children." *American Journal of Clinical Nutrition* 48, no. 2 (1988): 389–519.

Ruston, Roger. *Human Rights and the Image of God.* London: SCM Press, 2004.

Rutgers, L. V, M. van Strydonck, M. Boudin, and C. van der Linde, "Stable Isotope Data from the Early Christian Catacombs of Ancient Rome: New Insights into the Dietary Habits of Rome's Early Christians." *Journal of Archaeological Science* 36 (2009): 1127–34.

Rutgers, Leonard V. "Catacombs and Health." In *Children and Family in Late Antiquity: Life, Death and Interaction,* edited by Christian Laes, Katariina Mustakallio, and Ville Vuolanto. Leuven: Peeters, in press.

Ryan, Colleen. *Beyers Naudé: Pilgrimage of Faith.* Grand Rapids: Eerdmans, 1990.

Sachedina, Abdulaziz. *Islam and the Challenge of Human Rights.* New York: Oxford University Press, 2009.

Santiago, Rolando L. "Faith-Based Organizations and Public Health." In *Igniting the Power of Community: The Role of CBOs and NGOs in Global Public Health,* edited by P. A. Gaist, 93–108. New York: Springer, 2010.

Satlow, Michael, ed. *The Gift in Antiquity.* The Ancient World: Comparative Histories. Malden, MA: Wiley-Blackwell, 2013.

Schmid, Barbara, Elizabeth Thomas, Jill Olivier, and James R. Cochrane. *The Contribution of Religious Entities to Health in*

Sub-Saharan Africa. Study commissioned by Bill & Melinda Gates Foundation. Cape Town: ARHAP, 2008.

Schroeder, C. Paul, trans. *St. Basil the Great: On Social Justice.* Popular Patristic Series. Crestwood, NY: St. Vladimir's Seminary Press, 2009.

Schwarz, Timothy T. *Travesty in Haiti: A True Account of Christian Missions, Orphanages, Food Aid, Fraud, and Drug Trafficking.* Lexington, KY: BookSurge Publishing, 2008.

Sen, Amartya. *The Idea of Justice.* Cambridge, MA: Harvard University Press, 2009.

Shah, Rebecca Samuel and Timothy Samuel Shah. "How Evangelicalism—including Pentecostalism—Helps the Poor: The Role of Spiritual Capital." In: *The Hidden Form of Capital: Spiritual Influences in Societal Progress,* edited by Peter L. Berger and Gordon Redding, 61-90. London: Anthem Press, 2010.

Sheridan, Susan Guise. "New Life the Dead Receive: The Relationship between Human Remains and the Cultural Record for Byzantine St. Stephen's." *Revue Biblique* 106, no. 4 (1999): 574-611.

Si-Yu-Ki: Buddhist Records of the Western World, Translated from the Chinese of Hiuen Tsiang (AD 629). Translated by Samuel Beal. London: Trübner and Co., 1884, reprinted Delhi: Oriental Books Reprint Corp., 1969.

Singh, Prabhjot and Dave A. Chokshi. "Community Health Workers: A Local Solution to a Global Problem" [perspective]. *New England Journal of Medicine* 369 (September 5, 2013): 894-96.

Skolnik, Richard. *Global Health 101.* 2nd ed. Burlington, MA: Jones & Bartlett, 2012.

Sluga, Glenda. "René Cassin: *Les droits de l'homme* and the Universality of Human Rights, 1945-1966." In *Human Rights in the Twentieth Century,* edited by Stefan-Ludwig Hoffman, 107-24. New York: Cambridge University Press, 2010.

Snyder, Susanna. *Asylum-Seeking, Migration and Church.* Explorations in Practical, Pastoral and Empirical Theology. Farnham, UK, and Burlington, VT: Ashgate, 2012.

Spicker, Paul, ed. *The Origins of Modern Welfare: Juan-Luis Vives, De subventione pauperum, and City of Ypres, Forma subventionis pauperum.* Oxford: Peter Lang, 2010.

Stanford, John. *An Address Delivered in the Orphan Asylum, New York, February 5, 1822, on the Conflagration of the Orphan House in the City of Philadelphia on the 23rd of January.* New York: E. Conrad, 1822.

Stemmer, Juan E. Oribe. "Freight Rates in the Trade between Europe and South America, 1840–1914. *Journal of Latin American Studies* 21, no. 1 (1989): 23–59.

Stendahl, Krister. "Judgment and Mercy." In *The Context of Contemporary Theology: Essays in Honor of Paul Lehmann,* edited by Alexander J. McKelway and E. David Willis, 147–54. Atlanta: John Knox Press, 1974.

Sullivan, Susan Crawford. *Living Faith: Everyday Religion and Mothers in Poverty.* Chicago: University of Chicago Press, 2011.

Swidler, Ann and Susan Cotts Watkins. "'Teach a man to fish': The Sustainability Doctrine and Its Social Consequences." *World Development* 37, no. 7 (2009): 1182–96.

Tervalon, Melanie and Jann Murray-García. "Cultural Humility versus Cultural Competence: A Critical Distinction in Defining Physician Training Outcomes in Multicultural Education." *Journal of Health Care for the Poor and Underserved* 9, no. 2 (1998): 117–25.

Thomas, Liz, Barbara Schmid, Malibongwe Gwele, Rosemond Ngubo, and James R. Cochrane. *'Let us Embrace': The Role and Significance of an Integrated Faith-Based Initiative for HIV and AIDS.* Rondebosch, South Africa, and Atlanta, Georgia: African Religious Health Assets Programme, 2006.

Tobias, Phillip V. "Apartheid and Medical Education: The Training of Black Doctors in South Africa." *International Journal of Health Services* 13 (1983): 131–53.

Torvend, Samuel. *Luther and the Hungry Poor: Gathered Fragments.* Minneapolis: Fortress, 2008.

Trevitt, William, W. W. Dawson, Theo G. Wormley and John G. F. Holston. "Dr. Trevitt, From the Committee on the Mineral Waters of Ohio." *The Ohio Medical and Surgical Journal* 9, no. 4 (March 1, 1857): 283–96.

Turner, Victor and Edith. *Image and Pilgrimage in Christian Culture,* 2nd Edition. Columbia Classics in Religion. New York: Columbia University Press, 2011.

Tyndale, Wendy, ed. *Visions of Development: Faith-Based Initiatives.* Aldershot, UK: Ashgate, 2006.

Uvin, Peter. *Human Rights and Development.* Bloomfield, CT: Kumarian Press, 2004.

Virchow, Rudolf Carl. *Collected Essays on Public Health and Epidemiology,* Vol. 1, 204–319. Edited by L. J. Rather. Boston: Science History Publications, 1985.

Visser, Margaret. *The Gift of Thanks: The Roots and Rituals of Gratitude.* Boston: Houghton Mifflin Harcourt, 2009.

Vives, Juan-Luis. *De Subventione pauperum sive de humanis Necessitatibus.* Edited by C. Matheeussen and C. Fantazzi, with the assistance of J. De Landtsheer. Selected Works of J. L. Vives. Leiden: Brill, 2002.

Von Schubert, Katharine. *Checkpoints and Chances: Eyewitness Accounts from an Observer in Israel-Palestine.* London: Quaker Books, 2005.

Wagner, David. *The Poorhouse: America's Forgotten Institution.* Lanham, MD: Rowan and Littlefield, 2005.

Wandel, Lee Palmer. *Always Among Us: Images of the Poor in Zwingli's Zurich.* New York: Cambridge University Press, 1990.

Watkins, Susan Cotts and Ann Swidler. "Working Misunderstandings: Donors, Brokers, and Villagers in Africa's AIDS Industry." *Population and Development Review* 38 (Suppl.) (2012): 197–218.

Watters, Thomas, Thomas William Rhys Davids, Stephen Wootton Bushell, and Vincent Arthur Smith. *On Yuan Chwang's Travels in India, 629–645 AD.* Oriental Translation Fund New Series 14. London: Royal Asiatic Society, 1904.

Weinfeld, Moshe. *Social Justice in Ancient Israel and in the Ancient Near East.* Publications of the Perry Foundation for Biblical Research in the Hebrew University of Jerusalem. Jerusalem and Minneapolis: Magnes Press and Fortress Press, 1995.

Whaites, Alan. "Pursuing Partnership: World Vision and the Ideology of Development—A Case Study." *Development in Practice* 9, no. 4 (1999): 410–23.

Wilkinson-Maposa, Susan and Alan Fowler. *The Poor Philanthropist II: New Approaches to Sustainable Development.* Cape Town: Southern Africa-United States Center for Leadership and Public Values, 2009.

Wilkinson-Maposa, Susan for the Community Grantmaking and Social Investment Programme, Southern Africa-United States Centre for Leadership and Public Values. *The Poor Philanthropist III: A Practice-Relevant Guide for Community Philanthropy.* Cape Town: Southern Africa-United States Center for Leadership and Public Values, 2009.

Wilkinson-Maposa, Susan, Alan Fowler, Ceri Oliver-Evans, and Chao F.N. Mulenga. *The Poor Philanthropist: How and Why the Poor Help Each Other.* Cape Town, South Africa: UCT Graduate School of Business, 2006.

Winter, Jay. "Rene Cassin and the Alliance Israelite Universelle." *Modern Judaism* 32, no. 1 (2012): 1–21.

Woll, Allen L. "History Textbooks and the Secularization of Chilean Society, 1840–1890. *Journal of Latin American Studies* 7, no. 1 (1975): 23–43.

Wolterstorff, Nicholas P. *Journey Toward Justice: Personal Encounters in the Global South.* Grand Rapids, MI: BakerAcademic, 2013.

Wolterstorff, Nicholas. *Justice in Love.* Emory University Studies in Law and Religion. Grand Rapids: Eerdmans, 2011.

Wolterstorff, Nicholas. "The Way to Justice: How My Mind Has Changed." *Christian Century* 126, no. 24 (2009): 26–30.

Wolterstorff, Nicholas. *Hearing the Call: Liturgy, Justice, Church, and World.* Edited by Mark R. Gornik and Gregory Thompson. Grand Rapids: Eerdmans, 2011.

Wolterstorff, Nicholas. *Justice: Rights and Wrongs.* Princeton: Princeton University Press, 2008.

Woodcock, Andrew. "Jacques Maritain, Natural Law and the Universal Declaration of Human Rights." *Journal of the History of International Law* 8 (2006): 245–66.

Wooley, Charles F. and Barbara A. Van Brimmer. *The Second Blessing: Columbus Medicine and Health-The Early Years.* South Egremont, MA: Science International Corporation, 2006.

Yamin, Alicia Ely and Siri Gloppen, eds. *Litigating Health Rights: Can Courts Bring More Justice to Health?* Cambridge, MA: Harvard University Press, 2011.

Yamin, Alicia Ely. *Power and Suffering: Human Rights-Based Approaches to Health and Why They Matter.* Philadelphia: University of Pennsylvania Press, forthcoming.

Yamin, Alicia Ely. "Reflections on Defining, Understanding and Measuring Poverty in Terms of Violations of Economic and Social Rights Under International Law." *Georgetown Journal on Fighting Poverty* 4 (1997): 273–307.

Yamin, Alicia Ely. "The Future in the Mirror: Constructing and De-Constructing Strategies for the Defense and Promotion of Economic, Social and Cultural Rights." *Human Rights Quarterly* 27, no. 3 (2005): 1200–44.

Yamin, Alicia Ely. "The Right to Health under International Law and Its Relevance to the United States." *American Journal of Public Health* 95, no. 7 (2005): 1156–61.

Yamin, Alicia Ely. "Toward Transformative Accountability: A Proposal for Rights-Based Approaches to Fulfilling Maternal Health Obligations." *Sur: An International Journal* 7 (2010): 95–122.

Young, Katharine G. "The Minimum Core of Economic and Social Rights: A Concept in Search of Content." *Yale Journal of International Law* 33 (2008): 113–75.

Ziegler, Jean, Christophe Golay, Claire Mahon, Sally-Anne Way. *The Fight for the Right to Food: Lessons Learned.* Geneva: Palgrave Macmillan, 2011.

Zuniga, José, Stephen P. Marks, and Lawrence O. Gostin, eds. *Advancing the Human Right to Health.* New York: Oxford University Press, 2013.

INDEX

Page numbers in italics refer to figures and tables